PRESCRIBING
CHANGE

HOW TO MAKE CONNECTIONS, INFLUENCE DECISIONS AND GET PATIENTS TO BUY INTO CHANGE

STEVE VARGO, OD, MBA

Steve Vargo, OD, MBA

Optometric Practice Management Consultant

www.drstevevargo.com

© 2020 by Dr. Steve Vargo

All rights reserved.

Contents

Introduction

Why do you want to be an optometrist?

I was 23 years old, and that's the question I was asked as part of the interview process for acceptance to optometry school. If you're a doctor or healthcare provider, I assume you've been asked a similar question pertaining to your specialty.

I can't recall my exact answer (23 was a long time ago), but I do recall mentioning my desire to help others. I wanted a career that allowed me to improve people's lives. Whether you chose optometry, dentistry, chiropractic, nutritionist, massage therapy, or any other healthcare specialty, we probably all share the same desire to help others.

I guess that was the right answer, because not too long after I received an acceptance letter to the Illinois College of Optometry and off to school I went! Over four years, our young brains were packed full of information about the human eye. Histology, pathology, optics, color vision, ocular disease, pharmacology, and the list goes on. The curriculum also included some "why do we have to know this to be an eye doctor" courses. Thankfully, I never had to treat an eye emergency that forced me to recall the 26 bones in the foot or recite from memory all the chemical reactions that take place in the Krebs cycle. Whew! On the positive side, no one can accuse us optometrists of not being well rounded.

After four years of education that included live clinical care, residencies, rotations, and then passing board exams (I passed mine with ease – on the second attempt), they dressed us up in the typical graduation garb and marched us through graduation. We were doctors, ready to start changing lives!

I'M A DOCTOR, DAMMIT!

Let's face it, once someone deems us worthy to stick a few letters after our name, we sometimes let it go to our heads. My first few years in practice I placed a lot of importance on my title. I assumed others did as well. Over the years many of us come to realize that in the grand scheme of things we're not *that* important, but prior to that level of self-awareness I recall being shocked at the behavior of many of my patients. In spite of all the life changing infor-mation I was sharing with patients about why they should follow my desired course of action or treatment plan; many weren't doing what I told them to do. The nerve of these people! Don't they know I'm a licensed doctor?

Somewhere along the way I realized I wasn't God, and people didn't have to do what I said. If you're a young doctor or healthcare professional and still struggling with this concept, I suggest you accept this reality sooner than later. Once you do, you can begin to stop depending so heavily on your knowledge to change people and begin exploring new ways to get people to ACT on the information you provide.

As I refer to "change" throughout this book, I'm referring to the process of getting people to do something different. The problem so many of us clinicians experience is that the patients hear our information but fail to apply it. They don't *change*. I'll make the case in later chapters that the influence doctors have over their patients is not what it once was. There are many reasons for that we'll get into later, but for now let's consider that merely sharing information with patients often fails to motivate change.

I read somewhere that if information was all it took, we would all be millionaires with six-pack abs. How many times have we received financial advice or fitness advice or some other form of advice and logged away the information but failed to act on it? We gained some newfound insight but didn't actually change anything.

This is a struggle many healthcare professionals experience. Are we *really* helping people or improving lives if people don't act on the information we provide? Education is important, but education combined with action is the only way to truly make an impact on the patients we serve.

So, how do we do that? That's the question I ultimately asked myself. One day, walking down aisle two at the grocery store looking for toothpaste, the answer hit me like a lightning bolt! I suddenly had complete clarity on how to get people to change!

Just kidding. That's not how these things usually work, and toothpaste is rarely in aisle two.

I did, however, start having serious questions about how to get people to do what I was recommending. I realized the impact I could make on others directly correlated with my ability to get them to act on the information I was providing. The days of having an ego and wanting to impress people with a lot of medical terminology were gone. I didn't become an eye doctor just to feed people information. I wanted to get back to the reason I chose to become an optometrist. I wanted to make a real impact. I wanted to help people!

SELLING PATIENTS ON CHANGE

Before we continue, I have a confession to make.

When I started writing this book, the original title was going to be something different. In fact, I had about two-thirds of this book completed before I decided to change the title.

Why the need for a confession? Well, if you're a healthcare professional, the title may have offended you. The original title was *Even Doctors are Salespeople.*

[Collective gasp!]

Before you send me nasty letters and emails, please allow me to explain. I didn't intend this to be a book about "selling," at least not in the traditional sense of exchanging goods and services for money. While many healthcare specialties do sell products and services, I'm sensitive to the notion that many doctors and healthcare professionals prefer to distance themselves from the actual practice of selling. Optometrists, for example, will often tell you that their opticians are the ones who do the selling, even though the doctor may be discussing eye care products during the examination. That inspired the title of my previous book, *But I Don't Sell.*

But, do you sell?

I'm going to make an argument in this book that not only proves you do sell, but also reinforces why you need to get better at it!

"But I DON'T sell!" you adamantly proclaim.

Ahh, but you do, and you do it quite frequently. You sell patients on change! Start exercising. Take your contact lenses out at night. Start taking nutritional supplements. Lose weight. Stop smoking. Start wearing sunglasses outdoors. Whatever healthcare occupation you work in, you are constantly attempting to get people to change. This usually involves something intended to benefit their health or lifestyle.

For now, let's put aside the concept of selling products and services, the topic of most books on selling. Let's focus on a different aspect of selling that often goes unnoticed. As healthcare professionals, there's a lot we can learn and apply from good salespeople. A good salesperson gets us to *change* something that benefits us. If a prospect doesn't do anything with the information that the salesperson provides, how effective is that salesperson? How much of an impact did that salesperson have on the prospective customer if the customer did not change anything?

We can apply the same thinking to patient care. How much of an impact do we have on the lives of our patients if they don't act on the information we are providing? Considering many people are slow to embrace change, is it fair to say you must "sell" patients on change?

"Sure, I suppose," you're thinking. "That's why I thoroughly educate all my patients on my recommendations."

Umm, yeah. Let's talk about that.

How can I say this in a nice way? Maybe I'll just go the direct route. It's not working!

I'm not suggesting it never works, nor am I suggesting education is not a critical aspect of patient care, but clinicians are increasingly faced with patients who don't do what they are being told to do. You educate on why they need to lose weight, and the patient returns the following year 10 pounds heavier. Stop smoking! They return for their next exam with a pack of Marlboro Lights in their shirt pocket. You recommend additional testing to assess the patient's risk for disease, and the patient says, "Maybe next time."

In many cases, patients are forgoing even more urgent medical needs like annual physicals, dental cleanings and updated glasses prescriptions. A dentist friend of mine told me it's not uncommon for his patients to openly question the need for a yearly dental X-ray and suggest this is just a way for the dentist to make more money.

Clinicians, often in a moment of frustration, proclaim that patients just don't care. I don't believe that to be true. More likely, I think clinicians are running up against a basic principle of human nature - people are resistant to change!

Every day we are faced with having to make numerous choices and decisions. In the world of sales, we are constantly exposed to marketing messages and salespeople attempting to influence our purchasing decisions. Relative to the number of messages and attempts we are exposed to, most of the time we don't make any decision at all. We go about our lives not doing anything differently. Nothing changes!

The same applies to people's health. Every day we have choices and decisions we must make regarding our health. In the year 2020, there is no shortage of information. Thanks to the Internet, there is also no shortage of access to information. People know they need to lose weight and eat better and stop smoking and get an annual physical and floss every day and get more sleep and protect their eyes from the sun and on and on. They know this, but they are slow to change. Doctors think more "information" is the answer, but as you may have observed and as I'll explain throughout the book, information alone often fails to inspire lasting change.

Your success as a clinician, and also your success on a financial level if your practice does sell products or services as treatment options, directly correlates with your ability to "sell" people on change. In the words of Albert Einstein, "Nothing happens until something moves."

Back to the original title, I struggled with that for a while. I thought it was catchy but considering the target audience for this book is healthcare professionals, I had concerns that an aversion to the word "selling" might be offensive to some. It's hard to explain your intent on the cover of a book and I certainly didn't want to offend people. Also, I'm no book marketing guru but that didn't seem like a great way to sell a book! Eventually I scrapped it in favor of *Prescribing Change*. And I'm glad I did, because that's what this book is about – getting people to change!

In spite of the title change, in the chapters ahead I will frequently refer to concepts around selling. In the preceding comments I wanted to be clear with my intent in using that word, so I hope you'll allow me to use that term without taking offense. As a practice management consultant for independent optometrists, I've had to better understand how to be successful on the retail side of eye care. My job involves helping private practice optometrists become more financially successful. Through the process of researching, observing and learning what made some practices more successful at selling than others, I began to recognize certain commonalities. Where some practices struggled with getting patients to follow their recommendations regarding eye wear products and services, others thrived in this area.

While not necessarily a lightning bolt in aisle two moment, I did have a revelation that led me down a path of exploring how the skills involved in selling could be applied to getting patients to change. Many of the doctors I worked with had a strong aversion to the term selling, but they were looking at it all wrong. They were holding on to the used car salesman stereotype. What they weren't seeing was the ability of a good salesperson to inspire change in someone. A good salesperson doesn't manipulate, a good salesperson **helps people get what they need**!

Boom! That's what I wanted. I'm assuming that's what you want too! So before we throw the baby (or in this case the proverbial pushy car salesman trying to put you in a 2016 Camry) out with the bath water, let's go on a journey to see if some of the positive aspects of selling can be applied to patient care. Let's explore how to make connections, influence decisions and get patients to "buy into" change. This will lead to happier and healthier patients, and also a sense among clinicians that they are truly making an impact in the lives of the patients they serve.

With that said, let's take a closer look at what selling is and how you can apply it to your interactions with patients in getting them to change.

NON-SALES SELLING

Some healthcare occupations do engage in a traditional form of selling. Optometrists, for example, sell eye care products. Obviously, that would be a fundamental activity involved in selling, but as healthcare professionals we are often required to sell people on our ideas, recommendations and actions we want them to take. In fact, we do a lot of non-sales selling. Every time we prescribe a course of treatment, persuade a noncompliant patient to stick to the plan, or attempt to convince someone that the remedy they found on a Google search may not be the best approach, we are engaged in non-sales selling.

According to a Gallup study, people spend 40 percent of their time in non-sales selling.[1] This involves persuading, influencing and changing behaviors. The people in the study indicated this was crucial to their professional success. Just because you have a few degrees hanging on a wall doesn't mean every patient will follow your professional recommendations. Non-sales selling does involve an exchange of information, but I will reiterate throughout this book that information alone does not improve patient's lives. If you're a healthcare professional and want to make a positive impact on people's lives, then something has to change!

While nearly every healthcare professional engages in some form of non-sales selling, there are also many healthcare practices that engage in traditional selling of goods and services. If you're an optometrist, you sell eye wear. If you're a fitness trainer, you sell training packages. If you're an orthodontist, you sell braces and orthodontic retainers and all the service components that are involved with teeth realignment.

In my experience working with optometrists, I find that many have such an aversion to "selling" that they will actually avoid conversations with patients that they should be having. I've heard numerous doctors and healthcare professionals distance themselves from any and all aspects of selling, but on many levels this will become a disservice to your patients if it prevents them from getting the information or treatment that they need. I'm referring mostly to doctors or healthcare professionals who sell a product or service (dentists, chiropractors, optometrists, fitness trainers, etc.) A reluctance to recommend or prescribe what's in the best interest of your patients or clients will not only prevent them from getting the best care, it may also prevent others from getting the best care.

Assuming you reinvest revenues and profits back into the business to continually upgrade your services (new technology, staff training, office upgrades, etc.), then operating a successful business that thrives and continues to grow will benefit ALL your patients. When you look at it this way, don't you want YOUR doctor to be successful?

LEANING IN VS. LEANING AWAY

Have you ever been approached by a stranger asking for money? How about a knock on the door from an unsolicited salesperson? Or that dreaded experience of purchasing a used car and having to deal with a pushy salesperson?

In these situations, we tend to lean away. This could be figuratively, where we find ourselves guarded and skeptical of everything the individual says and claims. There's a lack of trust. There's a sense of risk and danger in doing business with this individual. How much will this cost? What if the product does not live up to the claims? How long do I have to spend with this person? Sometimes the response is so strong, we literally find ourselves leaning away.

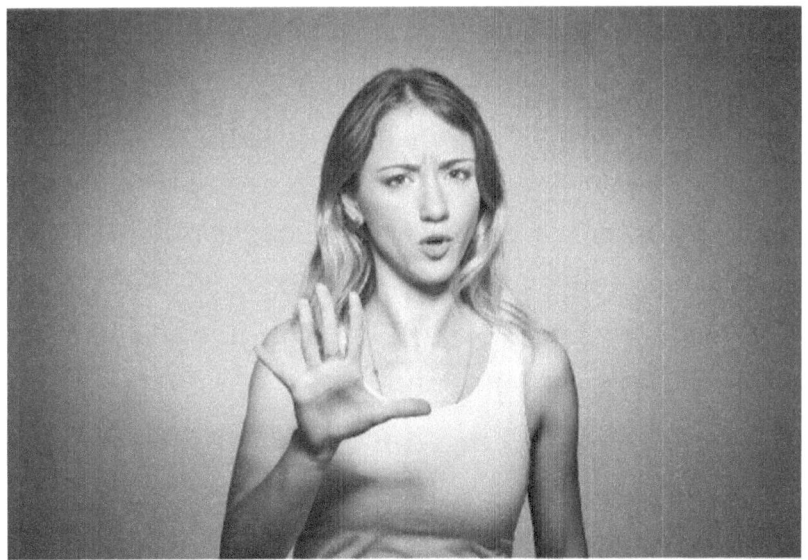

Herein lies one of the greatest challenges with getting another person to accept our offer when they are leaning away. We can't CONNECT with that person! They don't trust us. They don't believe us. They may not even like us! When we find ourselves leaning away from someone else, or they are leaning away from us, there is a poor connection.

On a personal level, think about a time when you were in a heated argument with someone. You pleaded your case, while the other person pleaded their case. How open were you to agreeing with the other person? How receptive was the other person to your comments? One of you may have even stated, "We're just not on the same page!" In other words, you were not connecting.

On a less contentious level, this scenario plays out every day in situations where we are attempting to get another person to buy a product, purchase a service, accept an idea, or follow a recommendation. Our level of success in these areas directly correlates with the degree to which someone is leaning in versus leaning away. When people are leaning away, they feel disconnected. When people feel disconnected from someone attempting to get them to take an action, their reaction will be resistance.

Let's describe a different scenario, one where:

- Another person showed a genuine interest in you.
- You found yourself letting down your guard and opening up about problems or challenges you were experiencing.
- You began to trust the other person.
- You wanted this person to help you!

Would it be fair to say that you developed a connection to the person described above? You were on the same wavelength. You wanted to hear what the person had to say. You were leaning in.

What I'm describing above is often the difference between someone who is successful at selling versus someone who isn't. Much of it comes down to intent. We'll get more into that in the coming chapters.

I want to bridge the gap between leaning in and leaning away. I want you to be effective at getting people to buy into your ideas and recommendation. I want your patients and clients to be more compliant with treatment plans. If you sell products or services, I want you to sell more of them. Not because you twisted someone's arm to buy something they don't want or need, but because you succeeded where others failed. Where others saw opportunity for themselves, you capitalized on an opportunity to help someone else get what they need.

This book is focused on change, but throughout this book I will make a strong case that to be successful at getting others to change requires a high level of influence, and the best way to gain influence over another person is to make a human connection.

It starts with connecting.

ABOUT THIS BOOK

Most of the content put forward in this book is based on a wealth of research conducted over the past seven decades. Even though I frequently consult optometric practices on ways to increase revenues and profits by selling more of the products and services they offer, I don't claim to be an expert on selling (at least not in the traditional sense). I would describe myself as someone who has a nerdy fascination with human behavior.

I'm fascinated with why people do what they do. I think this has served me well as a practice management consultant because I am less reactionary toward people's decisions and thought processes. I enjoy peeling back the layers and asking "Why?" Tell me more about your thought process or why you think this will work.

One of the greatest lessons I've learned over the years is that you have to understand people if you want to have an impact on their lives. It doesn't matter if I think or know I am right, my ability to motivate someone to take an action or change a behavior is mitigated if I can't connect with that person. Knowing this, I'm very aware that we can't connect over diverging ideas or thought processes.

The same applies to health care. We're always trying to get others to accept our ideas. Hopefully you're starting to see that even if you don't like the term "selling," we're always selling others!

As it turns out, if you want to be effective in this area, you must align your approach with how people process information and decisions. So often we violate this process, which only results in people leaning away. As mentioned, this can be obvious to the point someone physically creates more distance between themselves and you, or it can be more subtle in the form of a minor objection or a polite "I need some time to think about it."

This book incorporates a lot of research on behavioral psychology. If you want to be effective at motivating others to do something you want them to do, you have to understand these principles.

IT'S TIME TO C.O.N.N.E.C.T.

As I began to discover that a disconnect between healthcare providers and patients was a significant obstacle to getting them to accept our ideas and professional recommendations, I sought to find a method that allowed us to connect with the people we serve. I wanted this to be more than just ideas and theories that someone would read and find interesting but fail to execute on. I want the principles in this book to be actionable. Regardless of what field you are in, many top salespeople stick to a system. Without a system you are doomed to failure.

While healthcare professionals are less likely to identify as "salespeople," we are nonetheless in the business of having to sell. To do that effectively, we have to connect.

THE C.O.N.N.E.C.T. METHOD.

C – Curiosity is caring

O – Ouch! Where does it hurt?

N – No involvement. No commitment.

N – No time like showtime!

E – Earn trust

C – Conquer objections

T – Tell me what to do

The C.O.N.N.E.C.T. Method is a system, but it's not intended to be overly rigid. My goal is to provide direction and a framework that can be implemented in any practice, but there is room for creativity within each category. My suggestion is to follow the framework, but also do your own trial and error. Find out what approaches work best for you. Develop your own best practices. Ultimately, you will continually refine a system for your practice and patients that can be executed on by you and also taught to your employees. Once your employees begin to see how this approach is leading to happier and better served patients, they will give you the platform to help them.

We'll dig deeper into these topics in the following chapters, but please know that the ideas in this book are deeply grounded in human behavioral science. I'll apply concepts to the above topics that are scientifically proven to enhance your ability to be more persuasive and influential with people. These steps take people from leaning away to leaning in, getting them to not only understand the value of what you are proposing, but willing to take action based on their own ideas and beliefs.

Let me clearly state that this book is not about manipulation. In fact, it's the antithesis of manipulation. As healthcare professionals, it's incumbent on us to be influential and impactful in getting others to act on our recommendations, but OUR recommendation must align with THEIR wants and needs. Our role is not to manipulate, but rather guide people to the best solution. This is a subtle but critical distinction that will allow you to be much more effective in getting people to change.

If you *feel* like you are trying to get somebody else to take an action that mostly benefits you, then you will likely experience a feeling of psychological discomfort that prevents you from being effective. On a psychological level, it's relatively easy for most people to help others, but most of us are not comfortable in situations where we are asking others to do things that mostly benefit us. The key issue is one of intent. In the world of sales, this is a primary reason people don't trust salespeople. They don't trust their intent. When there's no trust, there's no connection. Without connection, you have little influence over people's decisions, whether that's purchasing a new car or starting an exercise program.

Before we dive into the C.O.N.N.E.C.T. Method, we first have to discuss how and why people process decisions, and why most of the time they're not even aware of it. That's the focus of the next chapter.

ABOUT ME (AND WHY I WROTE THIS BOOK)

After practicing optometry for 15 years, I made a career move to practice management consulting. The optometry profession may involve selling that's more overt than other healthcare professions (we literally sell eye care products), but the principles apply to many areas of health care. That's why I didn't limit the scope of this book to just eye care providers. I may draw upon more experiences involving optometry because that's the area I am most familiar with, but please know that the concepts put forward in this book are not unique to eye care.

That said, it didn't take me long as a practice management consultant to realize there was a true lack of selling skills in the eye care space, most notably around selling eye wear.

This was compounded by the reality that many doctors don't even like the term "selling." We're doctors! We don't sell!

In the same breath, these same doctors were complaining how difficult it was becoming to sell the products they offered. Consumers were increasingly seeking out cheaper alternatives in retail or big box environments, and the Internet was also becoming a major player. "How can I compete with that?" doctors complained.

In an attempt to remain competitive, many doctors began offering more services to enhance people's vision quality. Some examples are vision therapy that improves visual comfort while reading, sports vision training that trains your eye muscles to work better and enhances your athletic performance, and specialized contact lenses that reshape the cornea to allow clear vision without the need for surgery.

While these are all great services that would benefit many people, doctors were not always successful at getting people to commit to these treatment options. I'll think about it. Maybe next year. Do I really need this? As a result, many practices gave up on offering these services.

Since my role as a practice management consultant involved helping practice owners be more successful, I shifted my attention to how the doctor and staff could be more impactful in getting patients to comply with their recommendations.

My interest and curiosity led me to a wealth of research on neuroscience and human psychology. Eventually, it became evident that if you want to be successful at getting someone to do something, you have to understand how that person thinks and feels. People's brains are wired up to process information and make decisions in ways we fail to recognize when attempting to convince someone to purchase a product, take an action or accept an idea. Understanding these basic principles allows us to better connect with people. When you violate these principles, people will lean away. When you connect with someone, they lean in.

Now, let's take a look at how people make decisions.

CHAPTER ONE

The Science of Decision-Making

"We are not thinking machines that feel; rather,
we are feeling machines that think."
~ Antonio Damasio

"I have a dream"

Martin Luther King Jr. did not give the "I have a plan" speech, he gave the "I have a dream" speech. In the words of Rosalind Kennerson-Baty, a full-time lecturer in the communication studies department at Baylor University, "He had a masterful way of tugging at the head as well as the heart of those who wouldn't have been able to receive his messages."

This speech, delivered at a march on Washington in 1963, inadvertently set off a worldwide movement for racial emancipation. He delivered a message that changed the world.

"Don't give up. Don't ever give up."

These were the words delivered by legendary basketball coach Jim Valvano at a 1993 ESPY Awards speech that remains one of the most impactful moments in ESPN history. Valvano was nearing the end of his fight with cancer, and the speech was about never losing sight of what life is all about. "Think about it. If you laugh, you think, you cry, that's a full day," he said to a captivated audience. "That's a heck of a day. You do that seven days a week, you're gonna have something special."

The V foundation for Cancer Research, founded by ESPN and Valvano, has awarded over $200 million in cancer research grants nationwide.

"Ask not what your country can do for you; ask what you can do for your country."

Most people recognize these famous words from John F. Kennedy's inaugural address on January 20, 1961. What many people likely don't recall is the opening sentence. "We observe today not a victory of party, but a celebration of freedom — symbolizing an end, as well as a beginning — signifying renewal, as well as change."

Change. This is a common theme among these individuals. They wanted to change the way people think, act and feel. If they could do that, they were more likely to be successful in getting people to change the way they approached social injustice, terminal disease, or patriotism.

What was it about these individuals that made their message so captivating and memorable? What is it about great leaders and speakers that motivate others to want to change?

IT STARTS WITH CONNECTION

Change is hard. Even when we desire change, we often give up and resort back to our old ways. New Year's resolutions are a great example. Over half of New Year's resolutions are health or finance related, such as exercising, eating healthier, or getting out of financial debt. According to an article in the New York Post, 80 percent of people fail to keep their New Year's resolution, and research has shown that January 12th is the most common date for people to give up on their resolution.[2] Wow, 12 whole days! Pass the donuts.

If making change happen in our own lives is difficult, it should come as no surprise that getting others to change can be even more difficult. People resist change for all sorts of reasons. This includes patients who hear their doctor's suggestions, advice, and even warnings and fail to act on the information. So, what's the answer?

There is a formula I'll stress throughout this book, and it starts with making a connection. But not just any connection, the individuals mentioned above were able to connect with people on an emotional level. It's the same approach used by politicians, CEOs, coaches, and anyone else who aspired to have influence and create change.

Politicians rarely give you the logical reasons you should vote for them. They connect with you on an emotional level. That can be anger, fear, hope or other emotions that motivate action. If you were going to vote for another candidate, they want to change that. If you didn't intend to vote, they want to change that. If you don't care about politics, they want to change that. And they don't do it with facts and figures, they do it with emotion. If they are invoking facts and figures, it's usually to create an emotional reaction. Sorry, not to get on a political rant there, but it's true. Logic and reason are very often NOT the basis for our decisions, emotion is.

THE THREE-LAYERED BRAIN

But surely logic and reason are involved in people's decision-making, aren't they? After all, you're thinking, I spend a lot of time educating patients on all the logical reasons they should do what I tell them to do.

If they always do what you tell them to do, then you probably wouldn't have bought this book. If you aspire to have more influence with your patients, let's look at the neuroscience behind how people make decisions.

As you recall from neuroanatomy classes, the human brain has different layers with different functions. Layer one, the outer part of the brain, is the neocortex. This part of the brain is responsible for logic, analytical thoughts, facts and data, and the ability to understand and articulate language. This is also the area that allows us to recognize and judge situations and information. We'll call this the thinking brain.

Layer two, which lies under the neocortex, is the limbic system. This part of the brain is responsible for emotions, social interactions, memories and senses. This part of the brain stores not just what we experience, but how we *feel* about what we experience. Think of this as the feeling brain.

Layer three is the brain stem and cerebellum. This is the deepest layer, also known as the root brain. This part is responsible for safety, avoidance, balance, survival, and involuntary actions like breathing. We can refer to this as the instinctive brain.

Guess which part of the brain is responsible for decisions? A lot of the early research on this topic was focused on consumer psychology. Marketers were obviously interested in how and why people made purchase decisions. Initially, marketers and researchers thought the layers responsible for decisions were the neocortex (sometimes we make rational decisions) AND the limbic system (sometimes we make emotional decisions). We now know that nearly every decision we make begins as an emotional, instinctive decision. These decisions occur in the limbic system and root brain at a subconscious level, often without our conscious involvement. This sounds crazy, but most of our decisions are made seconds before we even become aware of them. Once the decision is made in these deeper parts of the brain, a message is sent to the outer, "thinking" part of our brain alerting us of the decision.

In a kind of spooky experiment, scientists at the Max Planck Institute for Human Cognitive and Brain Sciences attempted to predict the decisions of participants by scanning their brains. They were able to successfully predict decisions seven seconds before the participants were consciously aware of their decision. "Your decisions are strongly prepared by brain activity. By the time consciousness kicks in, most of the work has already been done," said study co-author John-Dylan Haynes.[3]

Let's relate this back to the world of selling, since the findings above have been widely applied in sales and marketing. When salespeople lead with facts and figures, this averts the decision-making part of the brain. The buyer is forced to use the neocortex to make a decision (the part of the brain responsible for skepticism and judgment). When you communicate this way, you're not only avoiding the part of the brain responsible for decision-making, you're talking to the part of the brain responsible for avoiding a decision.

Think about this as it applies to your interactions with patients. Is the information you provide connecting with the logical side of the patient's brain, or the emotional side? Are you directly engaging the decision-making part of the patient's brain, or the "thinking" part of the brain?

When you communicate in a way that evokes emotion, visualization and the other senses, you bypass the judgmental, skeptical neocortex and speak directly to the other layers. If you want to connect with someone in a way that's more likely to get them to make a decision that involves change, this is the part of the brain you need to connect with.

THE CONNECTION BETWEEN EMOTION AND DECISION MAKING

In 1995, Antonio Damasio, one of the world's leading neurologists, published *Descartes' Error*. For many years, science and even modern neuroscience had focused on the cognitive aspects of brain function. Emotions were largely disregarded prior to the publication of Damasio's book which challenged traditional ideas about the connection between emotions and rationality. Scientific discoveries were beginning to demonstrate that emotions were not just a luxury, but they played a significant role in decision-making and normal social behavior.

Imagine yourself as an intelligent, skilled and able-bodied individual. You're well aware of the day's news and have a fantastic memory of your life story. You test well on an IQ test and other areas of intelligence, and your long-term memory, short-term memory, language skills, perception and math skills are all present. And yet, the simplest decisions are paralyzing for you.

This morning you spent hours contemplating what to wear to work until your spouse finally picked out your clothes for you. At work you spent the entire afternoon trying to figure out how to categorize documents. Should it be by document size, date, or some other metric? When asked to make arrangements for a dinner meeting, you were unable to complete this task with only a few hours' notice. Even planning things weeks or months ahead is a challenge for you. You can think up numerous options but choosing among the various options is nearly impossible. This is not just an annoying character flaw. This is ruining your life.

While it may be hard to relate with the individual described above since you likely don't have this level of difficulty making simple decisions, this may be an accurate description of your life if you were unable to use emotions to process decisions.

In *Descartes' Error*, Damasio tells the story of a physician attempting to reschedule a patient for a follow-up exam.

> I suggested two alternative dates, both in the coming month and just a few days apart from each other. The patient pulled out his appointment book and began consulting the calendar. The behavior that ensued,

which was witnessed by several investigators, was remarkable. For the better part of a half-hour, the patient enumerated reasons for and against each of the two dates: previous engagements, proximity to other engagement, possible meteorological conditions, virtually anything that one could reasonably think about concerning a simple date. He was now walking us through a tiresome cost-benefit analysis, an endless outlining and fruitless comparison of options and possible consequences. It took enormous discipline to listen to all of this without pounding on the table and telling him to stop, but we finally did tell him, quietly, that he should come on the second of the alternative dates. His response was equally calm and prompt. He finally said, "That's fine." Back the appointment book went into his pocket, and then he was off.[4]

What's going on here is that this patient had suffered brain trauma that affected his ability to effectively use the part of the brain responsible for emotion. Thus, he was forced to rely on the parts of his brain responsible for conscious, logical thinking. This is not how the average person processes decisions!

What Damasio and other neuroscientists eventually came to realize was this: When emotion was impaired, so was decision-making.

Give careful consideration to this in your interactions with patients. We'll get more into the process of connecting with patients at a level that influences decisions, but for now know that your attempts to motivate change in people will often fail if you're only talking to the thinking side of their brain. It's not that the information isn't valuable, it's that information alone (without the involvement of the feeling brain) is often not enough to influence lasting change.

A MODERN-DAY INFLUENCER

Let's look at another kind of influencer. Are you familiar with the team "social media influencer"? If not, I suggest you Google that term, search out a few social media influencers, and go to their social media platforms (Instagram, YouTube, etc.). If you already know who these people are (and you're over 25 years old), you might need to spend a little less time on social media!

In many ways, these influencers follow the same formula as those mentioned at the beginning of this chapter, even if their message or purpose isn't the same. The formula is Connect-Influence-Change.

It starts with connecting, and social media is all about connections. Some of the top influencers have millions of followers. In most cases, these Internet superstars were extremely successful at connecting with people on an emotional level. Maybe they are funny, or create content that tugs at the heartstrings, or wildly eccentric, or travel to exotic destinations, or they do magic, or like my 13 year-old son told me when I asked why a certain Instagram celebrity was so popular – "She's really cute. Duh."

Social media, for all its annoyances, is a great lab for observing human behavior. Study some of the top influencers. Even if you don't "get it," observe the content and message and see if you agree that what they're sharing is connecting with people on a level that's more emotional that logical.

One social media influencer named Dahr Mann began creating videos a little over a year ago. He now has over 10 million followers on Facebook, Instagram, and YouTube, and his videos have been viewed over 3 billion times. I heard him being interviewed on a popular podcast where he talked about experimenting with different styles and formats. After a lot of trial and error and almost giving up, he ultimately discovered that the formula for success was to create content that connected with people on an emotional level. Considering the research in this area, we shouldn't be surprised at all by this!

I'm a few followers short of 10 million, but I have put a lot of content online as part of my job as a practice management consultant. I'm frequently sharing articles, information and tips. I find that the content that gets the most engagement is not the article on how to read a P&L

statement or a video discussing an HR policy. The content that gets the most engagement connects with people on an emotional level. My most watched video, by far, is a video of me holding a dusty iPod (yes, the original one that ONLY played music) talking about how your practice needs to innovate or become irrelevant, like this dusty iPod I'm holding.

What does the popularity of social media influencers have to do with change? Well, it's simple. They've connected with people, which gives them influence. Because they have influence, they get people to change. How do I know this? Because marketers and advertisers pay them to promote their products. Wear this shoe. Talk about this perfume. Listen to this band. Eat this protein bar. When you have influence, people pay attention. They are willing to consider change based on what you recommend.

Still not convinced? Let's talk money. According to Forbes, the top social media influencers can make thousands of dollars – per post! Rachel Brathen, a top fitness influencer, commands upwards of $25,000 for a sponsored social media post.[5] Not too shabby.

As a healthcare provider, you may never lead a civil rights movement, give a presidential inauguration speech, or become the next YouTube sensation, but your success is still tied to your ability to get people to change. You need to be able to influence people's actions and behaviors so they'll make the necessary changes to improve their health, or vision, or quality of life, or whatever it is that needs to change. It's through change that you impact lives. In the words of Tony Robbins, "By changing nothing, nothing changes."

THE ELEPHANT AND THE RIDER

In the bestselling book *Switch: How to Change Things When Change Is Hard*, Chip and Dan Heath describe the emotional versus logical sides of our brain and the effect of each on our decisions and actions.

- The logical, rational side analyzes our options and thinks long-term. This part of the brain is very good at self-control. The authors call it the "the rider," referring to a rider on the elephant described below.
- The emotional side of the brain feels pleasure, pain, love, empathy, and so on. It's more short-term oriented and seeks instant gratification. The authors call this "the elephant."

To summarize the analogy, most of us envision ourselves as the rider, in complete control of our actions and decisions and directing the path forward. What we fail to realize is that we're all riding around on a 12,000-pound elephant that's dragging us through life doing what it "feels" like doing.

While most of us like to think we are very much in constant control of our lives, in reality we go through much of our existence on autopilot. Depending on what time of the day you're reading this, you've probably already made hundreds if not thousands of small decisions today. If that seems like a lot, it's probably because you didn't have to exert much mental energy into those decisions. As discussed above, most of these decisions were made at a subconscious level. According to Harvard marketing professor and author Gerald Zaltman, ninety-five percent of our thoughts, emotions and learning occur without our conscious awareness.[6] And he's not the only expert who thinks this way; the 95 percent rule is used by many neuroscientists to estimate subconscious brain activity.

Imagine for a moment that you had to do a deep, logical analysis of every little decision you had to make throughout the day, from what to wear to work to what to eat for lunch. You would never get anything done! Our entire lives would be consumed by assessing options and weighing pros and cons.

The human brain has been described by scientists as a "cognitive miser." To allow us to live normal functioning lives, the brain has developed to preserve energy wherever possible. This is where the emotion – decision making connection comes in. The emotional side of our brain acts as a filter for many of our decisions. This doesn't always lead to good decisions or rational decisions, but nonetheless emotions play a huge role in our decision-making process.

Think of it this way. The logical side of our brain (the rider) knows we should live a healthy lifestyle. It knows we should change our diet and exercise regularly. The emotional side (the elephant) wants to eat a bowl of ice cream. Which side usually wins out?

As you go through your day, think about all the decisions, both big and small, that you make. Give thought to how many of those decisions were made as a result of a logical decision-making process and how many were made merely because you "felt like it" in the moment. As mentioned above, these can be good or bad decisions. You may have "felt" like going for a jog, or you may have "felt" like eating a donut. The point is that the elephant is a lot more powerful than the rider.

For our purposes as healthcare providers, it's very important to understand how people process decisions. Ultimately, the patient decides what to do with the information you provide, but when you speak the language of the decision-making part of the brain, you tip the scales in your favor that the patient will execute on the information you are providing.

ELEMENTS OF IMPACTFUL DECISIONS

Several years ago, I was seated at an airport waiting on my flight to board when two individuals sat down next to me and proceeded to have a conversation in a language I was unfamiliar with. As you might imagine, I wasn't particularly interested in this conversation given that I had no idea what they were talking about.

Suddenly, for no apparent reason, they both began speaking in English. These were two young men who were discussing a party they had attended over the weekend. Not only could I now understand what they were saying, but the story was quite interesting, and I found myself eavesdropping on their discussion.

I use this story as an example of how to get someone's attention. For our purposes, it's important that you get the attention of the decision-making part of the brain by speaking its language. If what your saying is not connecting with the more emotionally charged brain, it remains somewhat dormant. Since it's this part of the brain that has the strongest impact on people's decisions, it's important that we speak directly to this part of the brain using a language that it understands.

Research in neuroscience has identified five stimuli that speak to this part of the brain.[7] I'll briefly describe them here, and we'll take a deeper dive into these areas throughout the book.

1. Elicit emotional responses. When the brain stores memories in the limbic system, the emotions associated with these events are also stored. When people

communicate with each other, they constantly draw upon their past experiences, and the emotions that go along with these experiences. The subconscious uses these previous emotions to help drive decisions. This also explains why our decisions are not always logical or rational.

2. Be visual. Visual stimuli are processed by the brain faster than all other senses. The optic nerve is physically connected to the decision-making part of the brain and is 25 times faster than the auditory nerve. This is why they say a picture is worth a thousand words. What we SEE is closely tied to how we FEEL, and since we make decisions based on feelings, visuals are very powerful. Whenever possible, supplement your verbal claims with visuals.

3. Compare and contrast. Our brains are constantly comparing and contrasting. Good, better, best. Pain or gain. Safe or risky. This happens subconsciously in the limbic system and root brain. The brain wants to make quick, risk-free decisions and if the better choice is not obvious, the brain struggles to make a decision. If you want someone to make a change, increase the odds by contrasting the decision you want the patient to make with the alternative. Most people are not swayed by the scientific claims of weight loss supplements, they are swayed by the before and after picture.

4. Be experiential. As discussed, people make decisions based on feelings. Getting people to "feel" like they are experiencing something will strongly influence their decisions. Immerse the patient in the experience you want him or her to have. This is why salespeople often provide free trials, demos, test drives, etc. In health care, storytelling using 3rd party testimonials can accomplish this. What's more impactful, talking about the benefits of a procedure or sharing a story about a patient whose quality of life drastically improved after having the procedure?

5. Be egocentric. Our subconscious minds are always asking, "What's in it for me?" Even when we're being generous, the subconscious mind is wondering, "What do I get out of this?" This doesn't mean we can't be compassionate and empathetic, but the subconscious brain is wired for self-preservation. Always keep the focus on the other person and how the treatment, product or service you're prescribing will benefit them.

As you look at this list, many of the individuals mentioned above spoke directly to these areas. They connected with the emotional side of the brain, and thus were able to change hearts and minds and influence people's decisions.

Martin Luther King created a vision, or a visual. A visual doesn't have to be literal (like a picture); a visual can be communicated through story.

I have a dream that my four little children will one day live in a nation where they will not be judged by the color of their skin but by the content of their character. I have a dream ... one day right here in Alabama little black boys and black girls will be able to join hands with little white boys and white girls as sisters and brothers.

For the same reason you may have cried during a sad movie, even though you knew the characters were only actors, the subconscious brain has a difficult time distinguishing story from reality. Good storytellers create a visual in the mind of the listener.

John F. Kennedy used contrast in his inauguration address, mentioning beginning and end and contrasting the way things used to be versus the way they will be.

We observe today not a victory of party, but a celebration of freedom — symbolizing an end, as well as a beginning — signifying renewal, as well as change.

Politicians frequently speak in these terms. The old way versus the new way. The way things used to be versus how much better they are going to be. This creates contrast, which is a state of being strikingly different from something else. This is critically important for influencing decisions and getting people to change. The decision-making part of our brain needs assurance that the decision we are making is a good one, and clearly better than the alternative (which is often the decision to *not* change something). To quote Neil Peart (for all my fellow Rush fans), "If you choose not to decide, you still have made a choice."

While the ethics of politics are frequently called into question, if a politician's objective is to change minds, change voting behaviors, or influence decisions, they are wise to communicate this way. Lengthy presentations and bullet point slides listing all the great attributes of a candidate would leave voters confused over who the best candidate is, especially when the other candidates are offering the same presentation touting their own accolades.

This is why politicians typically attack their opponents with what is referred to as "smear campaigns." They need to create strong contrast between the options. We'll get more into the relevance of that later in the book, but for now just know that if you want to influence people's decisions, you have to demonstrate clear contrast between the options they have to choose from. Without contrast, people are often resistant to change and remain on the sidelines waiting for a compelling reason to act. This is why we need to "sell" patients on change.

For anyone who has lost or seen loved ones fight cancer, it would be difficult to watch Jim Valvano's "don't give up, don't ever give up" speech without being moved to tears.

Cancer can take away all my physical abilities. It cannot touch my mind, it cannot touch my heart, and it cannot touch my soul. Those three things are going to carry on forever.

While emotion played a part in all these scenarios, it was on full display during this speech at the 1993 ESPY Awards. People were moved to do something. The V Foundation has now raised millions of dollars to support the search for a cure.

In the world of sales and marketing, did you ever wonder why brands are so eager to get you to try their products? Free trials. Free samples. Download a trial offer. Would you like to take it for a test drive? They want you to experience the product. Proof always trumps claims, and it's very reassuring to the skeptical subconscious brain when it can see, touch and feel a product before committing to a purchase. The decision-making part of the brain is very risk-averse, and this helps it overcome that.

This is also why influencers are so valuable to companies and brands. If they can get an Instagram sensation to wear their line of clothes and rave about the comfort or a YouTube star to demo a product and write a positive review, that's almost as good as trying it out ourselves. That also plays into trust, which I devote an entire chapter to.

MAKE CHANGE HAPPEN

This is a book about change, and for people to change they need to make a decision to change. If I asked you why you chose to become a healthcare provider, would you respond by telling me you wanted to help people maintain their current health and quality of life? I suspect your aspirations are stronger than that. I assume you want to have a greater impact on the lives of your patients. For that to happen, something has to change.

The most important characteristic of emotions is that they push us toward action. In response to emotion, humans are compelled to do something.

If people heard Dr. King's speech and didn't change the way they felt or responded to social injustice, did the speech really have an impact?

If people heard Jim Valvano's speech at the ESPYs but failed to respond by *doing* something different, like donating time or money or even just reaching out to a friend or loved one struggling with medical issues, did the speech really have an impact, or was it just fleeting words soon to be forgotten?

When attempting to get someone to change, that person ultimately has to make a decision on whether or not to make that change. As discussed in this book, it's common for people to receive information but not act on it. In health care, this happens too often. I want to change that. I don't want your words to be quickly forgotten. I want you to make a real impact.

I wrote this book because I want you to have greater impact with the patients you serve. I want you to change lives, but before you can change someone else, you have to change yourself.

In the chapters ahead, I'll give you the information, tools, and resources to do that. The information I will share with you is based on many decades of research in behavioral psychology and neuroscience. When you understand how other people think, feel and make decisions, then and only then can you fully connect with them. Once you've connected, you will have more influence over your patient's decisions and ultimately make a greater impact in their lives by making change happen.

Now, let's C.O.N.N.E.C.T.

CHAPTER TWO

Curiosity is Caring

"People don't care how much you know until
they know how much you care."
~ Theodore Roosevelt

I'm an innately curious person. Some people like to share information about themselves, and there's nothing wrong with that, but I've always had more of an interest in learning about other people. What do you do for a living? What are your hobbies? How old are your kids?

Some people would refer to that as trivial chit chat, but the act of getting curious can greatly influence our ability to connect with others. What I've learned as a curious individual is that other people like to talk about themselves. Demonstrating curiosity simply gives them a platform to do that.

There is a term in optometry, which I assume in not unique to the eye care profession, called "prescribing from the chair." As the term implies, this is where a doctor reviews his or her recommendations in the exam room and prescribes the course of treatment. In optometry, this often involves the prescription of eye care products or services.

In my early days of practicing, I worked for a retail optical chain that wanted the employed optometrists to prescribe from the chair. The objective was tied to increasing sales of eye care products, specifically glasses and contact lenses. The recommended approach was very systematic. Here's the products we recommend, and we would like you to recommend these products to the patients you see.

There was something about this that felt awkward and uncomfortable. I also found it very difficult to get people to buy into my recommendations. The company I worked for never referred to this as "selling," but it sure felt like selling.

Years later, as I looked back on that experience, I believe I know exactly why it felt awkward and uncomfortable. The reason was because I had gotten away from curiosity. I was having one-sided conversations with people, giving them information and asking them to act on it. The reason many patients didn't act on the information was because even though I was a doctor, my influence over them was rather low. They respected my knowledge and credentials, but that alone wasn't enough to get people to change. The reason my influence was low is because I had failed to make a true connection.

Connection can be defined as a feeling of understanding and ease of communication between two or more people. The patient may have understood what I was saying, but I hadn't taken the time to fully understand the patient. Did the patient feel heard? Did the patient feel understood? There also wasn't much ease of communication, because I hadn't invited the patient to discuss his or her wants, needs and concerns. There was no true connection, just one individual listening to another.

If you want to make a connection with someone, you must show an interest in that person during your conversation. Research dating back to the 1970s suggests that people have conversations to accomplish some combination of two major goals: information exchange (learning) and impression management (liking). Healthcare professionals often focus on sharing information through patient education, but that is often one-sided and does not involve an "exchange" of information or create a likeable impression. Recent research shows that asking questions achieves both.[8]

Let's relate this to the world of selling, where someone is typically trying to get you to do something. This often involves purchasing a product or service. If the salesperson did not make an effort to fully understand your problems and concerns, you have a different impression of that individual versus a salesperson who demonstrated a high level of curiosity about you. The difference is obvious. One appears to be attempting to get you to do something that mostly benefits them, the other is engaged in helping you get something that mostly benefits you. In the latter scenario, trust and likeability are stronger, and that person has much more influence over your decisions.

Researchers at Harvard scrutinized thousands of conversations among people who were getting to know each other. The researchers told some people to ask many questions (at least nine in 15 minutes) and others to ask very few (no more than four in 15 minutes). Those who were randomly assigned to ask more questions were better liked by their conversation partners. When this experiment was conducted in a speed dating scenario, people were more willing to go on a second date with partners who asked more questions. Additional research at the London Business School and University of North Carolina found that job interviewees who excessively focus on selling themselves are less likely to be viewed as favorable as a candidate who asks more questions about the position.[8]

Sharing wisdom and knowledge is an important component of conversation, especially for healthcare professionals, but it's curiosity that leads to learning about people. Seeking to learn about others is an attractive quality that communicates we care about the other person's thoughts, feelings and concerns.

In Dale Carnegie's 1936 classic *How to Win Friends and Influence People,* Carnegie advises to "be a good listener."

More than 80 years later, most people still fail to heed this advice. The authors of the research mentioned above quickly arrived at a foundational insight as a result of their studies: People don't ask enough questions. According to their findings, one of the more common complaints people make after having a conversation is "I wish [s/he] had asked me more questions."

MY A-HA MOMENT

When I first started consulting, I worked for a company that was founded by a gentleman named Dr. Jerry Hayes. Dr. Hayes was well-known in the industry as a successful and business-savvy optometrist who had built several successful companies. To those who knew him on a personal level, he was also known for asking the question, "What's your a-ha moment?" He didn't even have to know you well. I once saw him ask a waitress this as she was taking our orders. He was genuinely curious about people.

It was easy to get caught off guard with this question, so whenever Dr. Hayes was visiting the office, we would all anticipate this question and scramble to come up with our a-ha moment. Typically, this would be some revelation we had learned or discovered since the last time we saw him. Sometimes these moments would come easily for us, other times we would struggle to think of something worthwhile to share.

After working for the company for one year, Dr. Hayes asked me his favorite question. "What was your biggest a-ha moment over the past year?"

I told him, without doubt, this was the easiest one to come up with. "My a-ha moment," I told him, "was that I learned to become a better listener." This was a lesson I had to learn the hard way.

When I first began consulting, I thought my job was to deliver solutions to problems. Here's what you need to do and how you need to do it. Technically, that is my job, but looking back I realize I was often too quick with solutions. In fact, my eagerness to jump in with solutions actually prevented me from providing the *best* solutions. What I mean is, I didn't take the time to fully understand the client or their unique problems.

A humbling moment for me in my early consulting days was when I interrupted a client as he was explaining an issue he was having in his practice. Having what I deemed to be all the information I needed, I proceeded to give him a detailed action plan that would resolve the problem he was experiencing. Or more appropriately, the problem I perceived he was experiencing. When I finished my detailed analysis and recommendations, I paused so he could ask any follow-up questions or perhaps praise me for flying in and saving the day for him and his practice. What I got, however; was a protracted period of awkward silence which was finally broken by him saying, "I already know that. That's not why I'm calling you."

That was the moment I realized, for me to be effective in this role I needed to become a better listener.

THE POWER OF QUESTIONS

Like many doctors and professionals, we can quickly get caught up in trying to impress people with our knowledge and wisdom. As tools for influencing people, that will only take you so far. Sharing what you know demonstrates knowledge. Understanding how people feel and letting them feel understood demonstrates empathy. Both are vitally important for inspiring change. There's a time to share, and there's a time to be quiet.

Questions allow for three critical components of making connections.

1. Relevance. Questions allow us to collect information necessary to deliver relevant messages. I dropped the ball with the client interaction described above. It's hard to connect with people when you don't fully understand their problems and concerns.

2. Attention. Questions allow us to capture and direct people's attention to what we need them to focus on. If we want to connect with someone (prospective client, patient sitting in the chair, someone you would like to date, etc.) we need to get their attention.

When was the last time you felt a connection with someone who wasn't paying attention to you?

3. Open knowledge gaps. Questions open knowledge gaps revealing what people don't know. The gaps where people have to think create curiosity about us and how we can help them solve their problems.

Relevance

Researchers estimate that most Americans are exposed to around 4,000 to 10,000 advertisements each day.[9] The majority of these are just background noise for most of us. TV and radio ads we don't pay attention to. Clutter in our mailbox. Spam in our inbox. Billboards passed on the highway with little attention given to the message. Sponsored ads appearing in our social media feeds that we scroll right past.

There are, however, times when an advertisement grabs our attention. We click on the ad, fill out the form requesting more information or call the phone number. Ask yourself what's different about these times? The simple answer: It was relevant to you!

On the topic of relevance, a friend of mine once told me about a recent eye exam he had with an optometrist. He proceeded to tell me how disappointed he was with the experience. When I asked what went wrong, he told me the doctor was very nice and thorough. The staff was very friendly. The office was high-tech with a lot of impressive technology. They also had a large, impressive selection of designer frames to choose from.

So, what was the problem?

"Well," he said, "They never asked me about ME!"

He said the doctor and staff made a lot of assumptions about what he needed, but never asked for his input. They recommended the *best* eye wear for all their patients, but my friend failed to see the value in all their recommendations, especially considering these tended to be the most expensive options.

My friend said that while they provided a lot of information, they never asked him about his occupation. Didn't ask about his hobbies. Never inquired about how often he used a computer or phone. There was no curiosity about him or his needs.

"They never asked me about me!"

I experienced a similar experience roaming the showroom floor at an industry convention. Since I no longer see patients, I didn't have much need for the products vendors were promoting, but that didn't stop vendors from attempting to sell me their products.

Stopping by a few booths, I was typically met with an eager salesperson anxious to tell me all about their revolutionary product and how my practice and patients would benefit.

At the same time, I was being handed brochures and literature that substantiated their claims. Of course, a business card was also presented so I could call with any questions and hopefully place an order.

Here's what they didn't know. I hadn't seen a single patient in over four years. Why didn't they know that? They never asked.

Had they asked, they would have learned that I transitioned from clinical care to practice management consulting and I work with an organization that forms strategic partnerships with other vendors in our industry. Vendors just like them! Perhaps we could have discussed synergies between our organizations and ways we could potentially partner, allowing them access to the thousands of doctors in our alliance. Potentially a great opportunity for both sides.

Unfortunately, that conversation never materialized, but thanks for the brochures.

In both scenarios above, the outcome may have been much different had there been fewer assumptions and more curiosity. Can you see how my friend might perceive that the optometry practice was mostly interested in making a sale? Can you see how I perceived the same thing walking the showroom floor at the convention? It's safe to say that my friend and I both felt that the other person or business did not care about us. There were no questions. There was no curiosity. There was no connection.

ME! ME! ME!

As discussed in the previous chapter, research has discovered that many of our decisions are made at a subconscious level by a part of the brain driven more by emotion than logic. This is an older, more primitive part of the brain that is mostly concerned about its own well-being and survival. We'll call this the "old brain," consisting of the limbic system and root brain. While most people are fully capable of displaying compassion and empathy toward others, that takes place in a different part of the brain. Therefore, if you want to influence decisions and inspire change in others, you need to focus on what's important to them.

When you understand the neuroscience, it becomes easier to understand how sharing information that is not relevant to the receiver is unlikely to lead to a connection. The old brain, scientifically proven to be responsible for most of our decisions, is asking "What's in it for me?" To answer that question, you must first get curious about what's important to that person.

There's something else that happens on a subconscious level when we perceive that someone cares more about their own interests than ours. It suddenly feels risky. We start to question the person's motives. We may even challenge their claims. We start to ask ourselves, "Do I really need all these features?" "What if this doesn't work like he says it will?" "Are they just trying to get more money out of me?"

When a decision feels risky, the old brain puts up a yield sign which can quickly become a stop sign if something doesn't change our perception of the situation. Without curiosity, we end up asking, "Do they even care?"

Asking good questions is all about executing the act of curiosity, and curiosity demonstrates that you care. When we perceive that someone doesn't care about us, and cares more about themselves, then there will not be a strong connection. We lean away. We don't buy, support or follow the advice of people we are leaning away from. There are exceptions to this of course, but I think we can agree this is not a sustainable model for a successful business or practice.

Asking good questions provides us with the information we need to later provide something extremely important for making a connection – relevant information!

Attention

In addition to getting people's attention by asking questions and tailoring your message to provide information relevant to the patient, questions also help you direct people's attention where you need it.

Have you ever attempted to deliver an important message to someone who appeared 1,000 miles away? They were there physically, but mentally their mind was elsewhere.

In the eye care world, I tell doctors that as much as they would like to believe that patients entering their practices are ecstatic about the prospect of receiving a thorough, comprehensive exam by a licensed eye care professional and then having the opportunity to pick out a new pair of frames from their expansive selection, I remind them that the average patient walking into their practice is not thinking about all of that. In case you hadn't noticed, people are distracted by events going on in their own lives. A fight with a spouse. Money problems. A child who's struggling in school. The list goes on. Unless you're a marriage counselor, financial advisor or school counselor, it may not be your job to fix these problems. However, for you to fix the problems you *are* being paid to; you must hijack people's attention!

Let me ask you a couple questions. What's the color of your car? You should be able to easily produce that answer. Next question, what did you eat for dinner last night? Again, that should be something you can easily answer. What I want you to do now is think about the color of your car and what you ate for dinner last night at the exact same time. I'll wait.

You can't do it, can you? When I ask a live audience to do this, I sometimes see people's eyes bouncing back and forth like they're watching a ping-pong match.

It's impossible for us to focus on more than one thought at a time. That's not to say we can't multitask or bounce quickly from one thought to another, but at any one moment in time we can only really be focusing on one thought.

The point of this exercise is to demonstrate how questions can be an effective tool for directing people to focus on what we need them to focus on. What were you thinking about right before I asked about the color of your car? It probably wasn't the color of your car, but the question steered your focus to that. When I asked what you had for dinner, did you continue to think about the color of your car? Probably not. I got you to think about a different topic.

While it's probably of little benefit for our purposes to direct people's attention to the color of their automobile or last night's spaghetti and meatballs, we do need to *temporarily* hijack people's attention while they are in our office or practice. A distracted patient is hard to connect with. If their focus is on something else, they won't be focused on you and your message.

In the next chapter we'll focus on how to construct questions that get people to not just reveal superficial information but get them to focus on their true pain points. These are the emotional triggers that motivate people to act on your professional advice. For now, just know that if your success as a healthcare professional involves getting other people to accept your ideas or change their behaviors, you absolutely must get their attention. Questions are a great tool for getting people's attention and redirecting their focus.

This is a good place to mention that for any healthcare professional who generates revenue off the sale of products or services, the patient or consumer's attention may very well be on price. In a typical optometric practice, once the eye exam is complete the patient enters the optical and becomes a "consumer." As a consumer, price is often a concern.

The tendency to give people more information hoping they will agree to pay more for a product or service is often met with resistance. This is their "logical" brain in action. People are less apt to be resistant when someone is asking them questions, and questions can effectively take people's focus off price and redirect it to their health and the benefits they'll acquire from investing in their health. This engages the "emotional" brain. Since the emotional brain drives decisions, this is where we want to steer their attention.

Information: *These lenses offer 99% protection from UVB and UVA rays.*

Question: *How will this affect you if your cataracts worsen and you're not able to continue driving?*

We live in the age of information. There's no shortage of people and businesses trying to sell us by sharing information. Based on marketing data mentioned earlier, much of it we ignore. Instead of just sharing information, get the other person curious about why they need you and how your solutions can help them. To do that, you need to open knowledge gaps.

Open knowledge gaps

Early in my optometry career I met with a financial advisor. This was the father of a friend of mine and I agreed to meet with him at the request of my friend. I already had a financial advisor I was working with and I felt that I had a solid grasp on the fundamentals of savings and retirement. But what the heck, no sense turning down a free meal!

The three of us decided to meet for lunch. My friend was late to arrive and I had never met his father, so the first five minutes of the meeting was his father and I standing awkwardly near the front entrance of Panera Bread wondering if the other person was the one we were meeting with. Indeed, we were. My friend finally arrived and made the introduction.

Once seated, my friend's father wasted no time in getting down to business. Basically, he peppered me with questions for thirty minutes. For someone I had never met, the questions become increasingly personal as he continued to ask them.

- How much money do you make?
- What kind of returns are you getting on your investments?

- How much do you have in savings?
- What is your plan for an unexpected emergency?
- What would you do if you couldn't work for more than 6 months?
- How much of your income do you donate?
- What do you do with the money that's left over?

Wow! To be honest, I was a little uncomfortable at first with the line of questioning. But I must admit, it was very effective in getting me to realize that I didn't know nearly as much about personal finances as I thought I did. Many of the important topics he raised I had not giving much thought to. I have a family. What *would* I do if I couldn't work for a long period of time? Could we afford that? Would we have to sell our house?

I recall driving home with a lot more questions than answers, but come to find out later that was exactly his goal. He used questions as a tool to get me to understand what I didn't know and why I needed someone with his expertise. It worked! I recall wanting to turn the car around. I had concerns and questions I wanted to ask him. I wanted to hear more of what he had to say. It wasn't the information that motivated me to want to make a change, it was the questions! His curiosity about me and the knowledge gaps he created caused me to be curious about how he could help me.

Stop and think about this for a moment. Imagine someone you're trying to persuade to do something is leaning away from you (literally or figuratively). How much success do you think you'll have in getting this person to follow your recommendations? We've all been there. We felt like we were wasting our time and theirs. If my friend's dad had come out of the gate pitching me on the suite of financial services his company offered, I would have likely been looking at my watch wondering how long this meeting was going to last. That's what we typically do when someone is giving us a sales pitch. We lean away.

Many times, people are not persuaded because they are not made properly curious. Curiosity is the first emotion we learn. It's the basis on which all our knowledge and experience is built. It's the impetus to change. There's no reason to change until people become curious about what other options exist.

Questions open knowledge gaps where people have to think. They have to ask themselves questions and come up with answers. This is one of the best ways to increase curiosity and also move people to the conclusions you desire. When it comes time to present a product, service or idea, people are generally more receptive when they are in a curious state of mind.

THE KNOW-IT-ALL PATIENT

Have you noticed that some patients don't need you? Because, you know, they looked it up on the Internet. We live in the information age and there is no shortage of information these days. For the healthcare consumer, that's not all bad. People have access to health information that was not accessible decades ago. It's generally good for people to be more involved and knowledgeable about their health. However, this is a good place to quote the phrase, "People don't know what they don't know."

In many ways, the challenge in getting your message across is not grounded in the other person's lack of knowledge, it has more to do with their willingness to hear your message. This is why sharing information and data too early in the process can be met with resistance. The same way your curiosity about the other person led you to learn about them, they need to become curious about you and what you can offer before they are willing to learn from you. Generate curiosity in other people about who you are, what you do and how you can help them! Giving people information gets mixed results. Getting people to *want* more information from you is a game changer.

Use questions to open knowledge gaps, and watch the person you're talking to go from leaning away to leaning in. Just like I did at Panera Bread.

DO THEY KNOW YOU EVEN CARE?

Being able to ask the right question is more important than producing the right answer. Questions uncover people's buried drives and what's important and relevant to them.

If we don't seek first to understand, it's less likely the solution or information we provide will connect with the other person. Asking a good question is about executing the act of curiosity.

The message we send when we don't ask enough questions is often that we are egocentric or apathetic. An over-eagerness to impress others with our knowledge, stories or ideas can come across as being self-absorbed. And if we never or rarely ask about others, this can be perceived as not caring. Neither of these perceptions make us likeable or trustworthy. It's difficult to form connections with people who perceive us as egotistic or apathetic. We lean away from people like this.

On a subconscious level, when someone else is genuinely curious about us, we lower our guard. We place more trust and confidence in that person. Our sense of risk lessens. They appear more likeable. We begin to lean in.

What's your a-ha moment? Such a simple question, but maybe the implications run deeper. Maybe Dr. Hayes' success as a doctor and businessman was not rooted in the question itself, but the fact that he cared enough to ask.

Be curious about the people you serve. How else will they know you care?

CHAPTER THREE

Ouch! Where Does It Hurt?

"If I had 60 minutes to solve a problem, I'd spend 55 minutes defining it, and 5 minutes solving it."

~ Albert Einstein

S uccessful businesses solve problems.

Years ago, I heard a successful entrepreneur say that. So simple, yet so true. In this chapter I want to focus on identifying people's true pain points. These are the problems that motivate people to take an action or change a behavior. Questions and curiosity will be a common theme of this chapter as it was the last, but we'll take it to the next level by using questions to uncover people's emotional triggers for change.

ELEVEN SECONDS

In the previous chapter I told the story of a friend who had a disappointing experience with his eye doctor. Overall, he was complimentary of the practice, but he felt that the doctor failed to make a connection. There was very little curiosity about my friend and his unique vision concerns. Had there been more curiosity about my friend, the doctor and staff would have learned about his frustration with having to wear glasses while playing softball on the weekend. He would love to try contact lenses again, but his previous experience was not great. He found them to be dry and uncomfortable, so he stopped wearing them. Had there been advancements in contact lens technology since he last wore them? Would they let him try contact lenses before committing to a purchase? He thought about bringing this up to the doctor but didn't get the chance.

You might be reading this and thinking, "But we always ask a lot of questions in our practice! We're healthcare professionals. We're trained to diagnose!"

In theory, that's accurate. But in reality, is it?

In one study researchers found that physicians interrupt the majority of patients in the first 11 seconds of the patient speaking, often preventing the patient from describing what brought them into the office. This study also found that only 26 percent of doctors even ask questions that invited patients to direct the focus of the conversation. [10]

Another study found that physicians tend to interrupt patients within 15 seconds of their beginning to speak at the outset of a visit, while uninterrupted patients tend to conclude their remarks in under a minute.[11]

Sadly, for the patient, the lesson here is to talk quick if you want your doctor to fully understand your health concerns. Very quick!

PEEL BACK THE LAYERS

The most important trait in selling may indeed be curiosity. Ironically, curiosity is not that prevalent. Instead of listening to people, we are quick to interrupt. Many people like to talk about themselves and try to impress others with their knowledge and insight. Even when we do ask questions, our curiosity often remains somewhat superficial. We ask questions up to a certain level and then we stop. We don't uncover the deeper concerns and problems that motivate people to take action or make a change.

How do we do that without being intrusive? I mentioned in the previous chapter that I felt a bit uncomfortable with the sensitive nature of questions that my friend's father was asking. In spite of that, it was very effective. I would suggest you execute some level of courage with asking questions. Below I'll propose an approach that allows you to quickly get people to volunteer more information about themselves, but also know that as healthcare professionals we tend to have more leniency than most other professions.

Patients expect us to ask a lot of questions, sometimes of a personal nature, so we can help them.

I like to think of questions like peeling back the layers of an onion. Try to think of the onion like a brain. The outer layers of the onion are analogous with the outer layer or neocortex of the brain which is responsible for logical and rational thoughts. This is obviously a very important part of the brain, but not the lead decision maker. We need to go deeper to connect with the decision-making part of the brain. Questions are the tool we use to accomplish that. Peel back the layers!

3 layers of questions

Layer 1 – thoughts, facts and details

Below are some examples of Layer 1 questions. These questions are designed to gain a basic understanding about the patient. While this book is applicable to any healthcare profession, I'll use eye care as an example since this is the space I am most familiar with.

How old are your glasses?

How often do you wear contact lenses?

Do you have sunglasses?

Tell me about any problems or concerns (yes, I realize this is not really a question)

Gathering thoughts, facts and details are very important. A doctor or medical professional must have a good understanding of this information to provide the best care. However; from the patient's standpoint there's no real emotional connection to this information. As you recall, we need to dig deeper with our questions to uncover the emotional reasons for making decisions. The questions above are engaging the logical, conscious part of the brain – the outer cortex. The old brain responsible for decision making is saying, "Wake me up when something interesting happens." If you want to be more influential with getting people to accept your professional advice, you need to connect your recommendations to their emotional motivators, not their logical ones. Peel back the layers!

Layer 2 – assessments and explanations

Layer 2 questions involve asking people to further assess and explain the information they provided from the Layer 1 questions. Below are a few examples.

Would you ever consider wearing contact lenses?

How does that problem affect you at work?

How did that condition impact your grandfather?

We've moved past basic thoughts, facts and details. We're not quite at the point where the patient is crying out, "Oh doctor, please help me! I'll do anything you ask!" but getting patients to open up about their emotional concerns regarding their vision and health is critical. I previously mentioned that if you want to be more influential with selling, you need to get the old brain's attention. Layer 2 questions allow us to say to the old brain, "Psst, you might want to pay attention to this."

The old brain doesn't obsess about facts and details. The old brain is very emotional, but the tradeoff is that it's not very intelligent. It struggles to process or make sense of words and abstract concepts. Medical information and clinical recommendations are not nearly as impactful without the old brain's involvement, and to get the old brain's attention the information you provide must be relevant. And I don't mean relevant to you! Sorry, but the old brain doesn't care about you. At all! It doesn't care how many years you trained to be a doctor, how much of a burden your student loan payments have been or whether or not your practice is successful. The old brain (yes, even the one in YOUR head) is very narcissistic. That being the case, appealing to its own self-interest is a very effective way to gain influence. What is the old brain most influenced by? Desire for gain and fear of loss!

Layer 3 – desire for gain, fear of loss

In the world of selling, desire for gain and fear of loss are considered the two dominant buying motivators. If we want patients to "buy" our ideas, recommendations or sometimes even products, it only makes sense that asking better questions should lead to the patient telling us their dominant buying motivators in their own words. Below are a few example questions that get patients to reveal this information.

If we could treat your dry eye, how would that impact you at work?

What impact would this condition have on your quality of life if it worsened?

Ah, there it is! The old brain. The decision maker. Nice to meet you! Thanks for joining us. You know that problem you've been so concerned about? We were just having a chat about ways we could help you.

If you can get people to reveal this level of information, you are no longer selling them, they are selling you! They are selling you on why they need you and your products or services. Telling someone else they need something is never as effective as them telling you they need something. Get people to sell you on what they hope to accomplish and why they scheduled an appointment with you.

It's also worth noting that this is how people *naturally* reveal information. When I consult with doctors, the initial conversations tend to be very business oriented. When I inquire why they hired a consultant and what they want to get out of our services, their answers focus on things like revenue growth, lowering accounts receivable or purchasing new technology. As the relationship grows, they feel more comfortable revealing the deeper reasons for wanting help. In my experience, I find that what most practice owners want is more personal time and/or less stress. Sure, more money is important, but often the desire for more money is to offset the lack of personal time and the overabundance of stress they are experiencing. Desire for gain. Fear of loss. It always comes down to those two. If you want to be influential with people, you need to get them to dig deep and reveal these motivators. Once someone has told you *what* they need (layer 1), try to get them to tell you *why* they need it (layer 3). Emotional motivators are typically attached to the why, not the what.

If you're a psychologist or mental health professional, you may have the benefit of numerous sessions with patients to uncover this information. For many other healthcare professionals who depend on this information to be more impactful, they may not have that much time. The layered question approach allows for quick access to this information. And remember, as healthcare professionals people want and expect us to fully understand their problems and concerns. We need to move the conversation beyond "What brings you in today?" and get to "How would your life be better if…?"

QUESTIONS INSPIRE ACTION

Often in the world of sales and marketing, salespeople will talk about asking persuasive questions. I think the most persuasive questions are the ones that inspire action. Consider this when you are deciding what questions to ask. What action do I want this person to take? Good questions can be a phenomenal tool for guiding someone toward a solution you feel is in their best interest.

Here's an example from my consulting work. Typically, when working with a new client I will ask about the doctor's goals for the practice. In fact, we offer what we call a "3-Year Growth Plan" for the client. My purpose in asking these questions is two-fold. First, I'm interested in whether they have clearly defined goals. If not, I want the questions to also serve as a tool for piquing their curiosity.

- What are your goals for the practice 3 years from now?
- What strategies will you implement to reach these goals?
- What challenges do you anticipate along the way?
- What additional resources will you need?
- How will you know when you've achieved success?

The gap where people have to think creates curiosity. They must ask themselves questions and come up with answers. Often the reason people are not persuaded is because they are not made properly curious. When people are in a curious state of mind, this a great time to bring up new ideas. There's no reason for people to change until they've become curious about what other options exist.

PRESENT AN OPPORTUNITY

According to research done by Forrester, 88 percent of consumers claim that salespeople do not understand their problems well enough to help them. Buyers believe only 25 percent of salespeople have an adequate understanding of their issue and needs.[12] I'm not certain how these numbers break down for healthcare professionals, but considering the statistics above showing how quick we are to interrupt patients before they've had ample opportunity to explain their problems and concerns, is it possible we're not always getting to the deeper, more emotional concerns people have about their health?

Hopefully, you're starting to see the value of curiosity and asking good questions. Good questions open up deep thinking. The financial advisor from the previous chapter could have just asked me some basic questions to gather thoughts, facts and details and then presented me with his suite of financial services, but he hadn't connected with me yet on a deeper level. I already had a financial advisor. Would his services really be that much better? His logical reasons for using his services would have been countered and challenged by my logical reasons for not using his services. This is the dynamic that plays out every day in sales scenarios, leaving people asking, "Why is it so difficult to get people to [use my service, buy a product, accept an idea, etc.]?"

When you understand the neuroscience of human behavior, you realize that almost nothing lights up the decision-making part of the brain like an OPPORTUNITY. Think about this in your own life and it makes perfect sense. For one person it's making more money. For another it's losing weight. For someone else it's finding a girlfriend. We're always seeking out an opportunity. There's always something we want or need and we are very drawn to people who can help us get it. Opportunities very much align with desire for gain and fear of loss. We are typically trying to fill a void with something we want or need that we don't currently have, or we are trying to avoid the loss of something we do not want to lose. This is why it's so important to uncover this information with questions. Where does it hurt?

EXTERNAL PROBLEMS VS. INTERNAL FRUSTRATIONS

Companies sell solutions to external problems. Car dealer-ships sell vehicles that allow people to get from point A to point B. Gyms sell memberships to people who want to lose weight or get in better shape. Optometry practices sell eye wear that allows people to see clearer.

Given the definitions above, can you see how all these products are substitutable? If my only goal is transportation, I can buy any car to accomplish that. If I want to get in better shape, I have numerous options for health clubs in my area. If my vison is blurry, I can go to any number of eye care practices in my town to purchase glasses or contact lenses.

What I'm describing above is the mindset than many consumers have. It's called the commodity mindset. Merriam-Webster defines commodity as "a mass-produced unspecialized product." Care to guess what people focus on when they're in a commodity mindset? If you guessed price, you would be correct!

To complete the statement above, companies sell solutions to external problems, but consumers buy solutions to internal frustrations.

One of the top reasons we lack influence with people who could benefit from our products and services is that our questions only get people to reveal superficial information. As it turns out, many automobile consumers do not purchase a car based solely on transportation, but rather how the car makes them feel. Sure, most of us consider factors such as gas mileage and safety features, but these are layer 1 motivators. On a deeper level, the individual may have been embarrassed about the condition of his previous car or wants to make an impression with his friends and neighbors by driving an expensive luxury model. The individual considering a gym membership may outwardly declare he wants to lose weight, but inwardly he's struggling in his dating life and feels this will help him get a girlfriend. The person who shows up for an eye exam may write "need new glasses" on her intake form, but the internal frustration could be peripheral distortion with her progressive lenses that is affecting her golf game.

On a personal level, I've visited two chiropractors in my life. Both times, my reason for the visit was lower back pain. That was the external problem I was having. My internal frustration was the impact it was having on my lifestyle. The pain had a significant impact on my mobility, but what impacted me on a deeper level was not being able to play with my young kids. They were too young to understand why dad couldn't chase them around or throw them in the air. The physical pain hurt. The emotional pain sucked!

I mentioned that I saw two different chiropractors for this condition. One focused mostly on the physical pain. He never really inquired about the impact it was having on my personal life, work life, and so on. We never discussed it. The other doctor took the time to peel back the layers. As a result, at one appointment I had to pause and take a deep breath because I was getting so frustrated talking about the impact it was having for me at home. He cared enough to ask, so I felt comfortable opening up.

Care to guess which chiropractor I kept seeing? Both were qualified to fix my back, but only one made a connection.

Dentists! I don't want to leave you out. About ten years ago I got braces. I won't reveal my age here, but just know that ten years ago I was not a teenager! My dental hygienist suggested it. My first thought was, "You can't be serious!" Not only was I not a kid, but I was a practicing optometrist who had to work with the public. This wasn't the kind of job where you can hide behind a computer. I had to talk and interact with people every day. Braces?

Initially, my dental hygienist gave me a lot of logical reasons for getting braces. Most of these reasons were clinical in nature. I had a narrow upper jaw and my upper and lower teeth did not align as they were supposed to. This also created a lot of crowding with my teeth that had worsened over the years. She told me this could eventually lead to problems with headaches, gum disease and even the loss of teeth. Oddly enough, that was not a strong motivator for me to commit the next few years of my life to braces. I suppose I figured I would just deal with this when I was older.

At one point I interjected, "I actually *have* thought about getting braces." What she said after that changed the dynamic of the conversation. She said, "Why have YOU thought about getting braces?"

I paused for a moment, and then told her that for my entire adult life and much of my adolescent life, whenever someone would take my picture, I never felt comfortable smiling. If I were to laugh hard, you would have probably seen me cover my mouth with my hand or turn my head away.

That was it. That was my desire for gain / fear of loss. It's not that I didn't care about gum disease or tooth loss, that just wasn't a strong motivator for me to make this change in my 30s. I wanted to be able to smile and laugh without feeling self-conscious.

Ultimately, I agreed to make an appointment with an orthodontist and proceed with braces. If my hygienist never asked the question, it's unlikely I would have made the appointment. If the conversation never uncovered my emotional reasons for wanting to make this change, it's unlikely I would have followed through with the treatment.

The layered approach I proposed has been an effective tool for me in getting people to peel back the layers and reveal deeper information about themselves and their dominant motives for wanting to take an action or make a change.

If you can uncover that information and communicate to the person how you can help them, it's almost impossible to *not* form a connection with that individual. You have their old brain's attention, and it's clinging to your every word.

SHINE A SPOTLIGHT ON THE PROBLEM

What about people who don't claim to be having any significant problems?

For the patient or consumer, a problem is not a problem until it is recognized as such. In these situations, it can be helpful to provide valuable insight that opens the door to a conversation. The idea is to provide provocative insight around an area that is not only of interest to the other person, but also a problem you can help them solve.

As an example, I know from experience that staff management is a huge pain point for many practice owners. If I'm talking with a prospective client about the benefits of hiring a consultant and I'm not getting valuable feedback from my initial questions, I may move the conversation in a direction that shines a spotlight on potential problems. For example, "In my experience, managing employees is a top challenge for many practice owners. What has your experience been?"

When I was practicing optometry, here are some questions I would routinely ask when the patient was not forthcoming:

- A lot of computer users who wear contact lenses experience dryness and irritation when working. Have you experienced similar problems?

- We do see a higher prevalence of eye conditions like cataracts and macular degeneration with people who work outdoors. Is this a concern of yours?
- Many of our patients who wear this particular lens have complained of distorted peripheral vision. Have you had any issues with this?

As you start "peeling back the layers" with patients, I suggest you track responses for a period of time. Are there common problems and pain points that you consistently hear? Knowing this gives you more insight into the mind of the typical patient or consumer and helps you formulate questions that open the door to a conversation. Sometimes people can be very forthcoming with their problems without much work on your end. Other times you'll need to probe a bit to get the information.

In the end, it's possible that your questions lead you to discover that the person is not having any significant problems. That's ok too. The goal is not to manufacture pain points or twist someone's arm to do or buy something they don't want or need. The goal is to connect.

If people are walking out of your practice feeling they were "upsold," they may be feeling manipulated. If people walk out of your practice feeling like all their needs were not met, they may be feeling ignored. When people walk out of your practice feeling that you took the time to listen to and understand their individual needs and provided a solution that met or exceeded their expectations, they are likely feeling connected.

It's a long-held belief that top salespeople are great at problem solving. What matters more today is problem finding. Help people uncover challenges they may not even know they have.

As a healthcare professional, knowing what people need will only get you so far. Understanding how people *feel* will open a world of possibilities.

CHAPTER FOUR

No Involvement.
No Commitment.

"Without involvement, there is not commitment."

~ Stephen Covey

Early in my career I was attending a continuing education seminar where the speaker, an expert on glaucoma, was discussing various treatment options for glaucoma patients. At one point in the presentation, the speaker referenced a patient of his who had been noncompliant with his prescribed treatment. This led to a discussion with the patient about her various treatment options. He wanted to let her know that there were multiple options for treating her condition, but they needed to agree on one that would not only stop or contain further vision loss, but also one that that she would commit to sticking with.

While he was sharing this story, a hand went up in the audience. It was another doctor who was questioning the speaker's willingness to provide options to this patient when the current literature supported the current treatment as being the most efficacious.

The exchange volleyed back and forth a few times. As I recall, the speaker was patient and composed in his replies, but the audience member grew increasingly agitated. The speaker agreed that the current treatment plan may have been the most effective per current literature and studies, however it was not nearly as effective as it should be without the patient's compliance. His approach was to find an alternative treatment plan that the patient would commit to.

Eventually, the doctor in the audience angrily blurted out, "Who's the doctor here?"

DOCTOR KNOWS BEST

I'm aware there are times when a doctor or healthcare professional must insist on a specific treatment plan. In eye care for example, there are times when a patient's request for a less expensive generic medication is a reasonable request that can be accommodated. There are also times when a more severe condition significantly limits the options. The doctor in me felt the need to clarify that.

With that said, I want you to consider your gut reaction to the following scenario. Imagine your next patient walks into your exam room, sits down and begins telling you everything he wants regarding his care.

I'll paraphrase an actual patient of mine who said the following immediately after I introduced myself:

> *"Here's what I want doc. I don't need any fancy glasses; I just want what my insurance covers. I don't care if there's any glare, so don't try to sell me that no-glare coating. I also don't need bifocals! My last doctor tried to sell me those, but I just take my glasses off to read. I do fish and I need some good sunglasses. My fishing buddies told me to get polarized lenses. I think that's what they're called. I can't get my eyes dilated today because I don't have time, but I would like to know more about that test you do to check for macular degeneration. My grandfather had that and it got real bad. I worry about that."*

What was my reaction to this? Well, I admit I was a little put off. "I'm the doctor here," I was thinking. "I don't show up at your place of employment and tell you how to do your job!"

While this is probably not the most tactful way to communicate with your doctor, I use this story because despite this patient's somewhat brash approach, he did share something very valuable. He told me what's important to HIM!

Fortunately, the patient I discussed above is not representative of the typical patient I saw. Most were much more subtle and respectful. Then again, what good is subtle and respectful if the patient isn't going to follow your advice? Looking back, I find myself appreciating his candidness.

Most patients would have kept these thoughts to themselves. Most doctors would have made recommendations without fully understanding what's important and valuable to the patient. The result is a disconnect. No connection, no influence, no change. See how that works?

Our role as healthcare providers does involve informing and educating and sometimes redirecting people in their choices and preferences, but attempting to do this when the patient feels a disconnect is often met with resistance. Make a connection, and then you'll have greater influence. The goal of this book is change, and to do that consistently and effectively you must first establish a connection.

For now, I'm going to ask you to suspend your "doctor knows best" thinking and consider the following question:

Am I focusing more on what's important to me or the patient?

PATIENT-CENTERED CARE

There is a growing body of evidence that highlights the potential benefits of patient-centered care for clinical outcomes, patient's health and provider's financial performance. For example, several hospitals that encourage patient-centered care by paying greater attention to patient's needs and preferences have found that adverse events decrease, operating costs decrease, malpractice claims decline, length of stays are shorter, and the hospital's costs per case decline.[13,14]

Similarly, heart attack patients who did not receive patient-centered care were found to have worse long-term outcomes. Their overall health and likelihood of experiencing chest pains was higher than patients who received such care.[15] A study of patient-centered nursing interventions for cancer patients found that the interventions were correlated with improved patient self-representation, optimism, and sense of well-being.[16]

Despite numerous studies highlighting the benefits of patient-centered care and its correlations with better health outcomes and quality of life, studies have also concluded that patients often are insufficiently involved in care decisions. Fewer than half of patients receive clear information on the benefits and risks of treatment options, and fewer than half are satisfied with their level of control in medical decision making.[17]

Studies have found that patients and clinicians often have differing views on the importance of different heath goals and health care risks.[18] Other studies have found that physicians have inaccurate perceptions of their patient's health beliefs, often assuming what's important or relevant to the clinician is aligned with what's important to the patient.[19,20] When patients become an active participant in their care, this misperception improves. Unfortunately, not only are patients frequently not involved in their care, but they are often interrupted by their doctor before having an opportunity to fully express their concerns.

Do patients desire more control and involvement? According to Pew Research Center, 80 percent of Internet users now seek health information online, making this the third most popular Internet activity. Patients are also seeking information on diagnoses, tests and prescriptions to learn more after a doctor's appointment.[21]

As a healthcare professional, you would likely acknowledge that a primary role of yours is to educate and inform the patients that you treat. While this is certainly an important responsibility of healthcare providers, education and information alone does not have much impact on your patient's health and outcomes if it doesn't get the patient to act on the information.

All your patients who smoke know that smoking is bad for their health. Every patient of yours who is on multiple medications and overweight (barring factors outside their control) knows they need to lose weight and take better care of themselves. They've been told this by every doctor that they've seen. In eye care, we routinely tell people the risks of ultraviolet radiation to the eyes, only to watch many people decline the option to wear sunglasses.

For years medical professionals have operated under the premise that patients need information and instructions on what to do. While patient education is an extremely valuable component of patient care, it often proves to be an ineffective approach when patients are not active participants in their care.

Because you're an expert, most patients will politely agree with what you tell them, or at least give the appearance of agreeing. The question becomes, are patients committed to what you are asking them to do, or just politely bobbing their heads up and down to indicate they are hearing what you are saying?

THE HEAD NOD

Have you ever been in a situation where someone else was attempting to get you to do something or buy something and you found yourself nodding your head up and down while they were speaking? While your head movements were indicating "Yes", your internal voice was saying something like:

- How much longer am I going to have to listen to this person ramble on?
- What does any of this mean?
- What should I make for dinner tonight?

As a healthcare professional, have you ever experienced this from the opposite vantage point? You were highlighting the benefits of a medical product you offer or a treatment plan you recommend and the person you were speaking with was nodding his head up and down? You assumed this person agreed with everything you were saying and was eagerly ready to follow your advice. To your surprise, this person decided to forego your recommendations.

A common example of this in the eye care profession is the patient who listens intently to all the doctor's recommendations at the conclusion of the exam. "I'm prescribing glasses for everyday use with special lens features and also sunglasses to protect your eyes from UV radiation when spending time outdoors. I also see some problems from chronic dry eye likely exasperated by the amount of computer work that you do. I would like to see you back next week for some additional testing to determine the best course of treatment for that condition," the doctor states as the patient nods his head up and down in a series of affirmative head nods.

Later that day, your optician informs you the patient decided to order just one pair of glasses that were covered by his insurance and mentioned he would call back to schedule the additional testing. The following week you look at your schedule and do not see the patient's name. When you inquire, the staff informs you that the patient did call back, but only to inform your office that he found the glasses somewhere cheaper and would like to cancel his order.

Eventually I came to realize that the head nod is not an agreement nor is it a commitment, it is simply a polite acknowledgement that someone is listening. This person has not agreed to ANYTHING yet! This raises the question, how do you get someone to not just listen to what you're saying, but actually commit to what you're asking them to do?

THE INVOLVED VS. DIRECTED PATIENT

Chapters 2 and 3 focused heavily on asking good questions and uncovering the pain points and emotional triggers that motivate people to act. Once we peel back the layers and expose someone's desire for gain or fear of loss, we can present ideas and solutions relevant to that individual's wants and needs. To be influential with people, we need to create opportunities for them!

We also presented the analogy of the rider and the elephant. Even though the elephant (the subconscious, emotional part of our brain) is taking us on a daily expedition through life without much conscious input from us and also making a lot of our decisions for us without our "logical" involvement, we still like to feel like we are in control.

Consider how you feel when you step on an airplane versus driving a car. According to the CDC, more than 32,000 people are killed and 2 million are injured each year from motor vehicle crashes.[22] While catastrophic, airplane fatalities are extremely rare, while automobile accidents happen every day. Nevertheless, how many people would admit they are much more apprehensive about boarding an airplane vs. driving a car?

The issue is one of control. When we're not in control of a situation, it feels uncomfortable. We like to be involved.

In the last chapter of this book I will somewhat contradict that last statement but with one caveat. We are often happy to hand over control to someone we fully trust to advise us and guide us to the best decisions, whether it's soliciting a restaurant recommendation from a friend, agreeing to expensive car repairs when recommended by a trusted mechanic, or following the treatment regimen prescribed by your trusted family doctor.

Let's assume at this stage of the book that you are not there yet. That level of trust must be earned, and that's what this book is about.

But I'm a doctor! Doesn't everybody trust doctors?

Ever heard the phrase "second opinion"?

THE DISCONNECT

Doctor: *"Ms. Smith, we got the results of your blood work back and I have some concerns about your cholesterol levels. We've discussed your cholesterol levels in the past and as you know I've been monitoring your levels. Your LDL, as you may recall that's the "bad cholesterol," has increased since last year and I believe it's time to intervene. I would like to put you on what's called a statin drug. You'll take this once a day, and the effects can be quite profound. We should start to see major changes in your cholesterol levels within two to four weeks."*

Ms. Smith: Head bobs up and down while doctor speaks.

Interactions like this take place in healthcare clinics every day. Chronic diseases like high cholesterol are extremely common and often treated with medications like statin drugs.

As the doctor talks and the patient head nods, the implication is that both parties are on the same page. However; that's not the case at all. As is often the case, patients remain quiet with their concerns and objections because they are reluctant to challenge or second-guess their doctor. Let's take a look at the inner voice of Ms. Smith.

Statins? Oh my! I've heard a lot of bad things about those. My neighbor took those for a while and had a lot of side effects. I think her doctor took her off them. I wonder if I should get another opinion.

Do you see the disconnect here? Was Ms. Smith given an opportunity to be a participant in her care, or was it directed *at* her? Do you think Ms. Smith will be more likely or less likely to be compliant with treatment if she leaves the office with these unaddressed concerns and objections?

While the scenario above was fictitious, the reality was not. Patients often bring a different perspective to the encounter than clinicians, and patients who are not involved in their healthcare decisions are more likely to regret their choices and less likely to stick to the treatment regimens.[23]

Interestingly, studies have found that patients on statin drugs are indeed far more likely than their clinician to initiate the discussion of symptoms potentially related to the prescription.[24]

What about patients who refrain from expressing their concerns? What about patients who feel their doctor is busy and doesn't have time to listen to their concerns? What about patients who feel their concerns were dismissed? What about patients who don't feel involved?

Whether we admit it or not, healthcare professionals are often guilty of trying to "sell" patients on treatment strategies that we feel are in their best interest without considering the patient's preferences, values and life circumstances. If you feel that shared decision-making and a more patient-centric approach could lead to better outcomes, then there's a word we need to start using more.

IT'S ALL ABOUT "YOU"

In the book Presentations Plus by David Peoples, he referenced a study that listed the 12 most persuasive words in the English language.[25] There are other studies that sought to find this information as well, and while there are some variations among these lists, there is one word that consistently appears at the top. That word is "You."

The reason I focused the early chapters on asking questions and uncovering the patient's most urgent pains and concerns is so we could tie solutions and outcomes directly to things that are important to the patient.

- "What this means to YOU is…"
- "Why this is important for YOU is…"
- "One of the things I heard YOU say is…"

For those of you reading this and still thinking, "Who's the doctor here?", I get it. Let me reassure you that the objective here is not to let patients completely dictate their care, but rather to guide the patient toward the best treatment options taking into consideration what's important to them. Just because "doctor knows best" does not necessarily mean the patient will follow our professional advice.

Instead of challenging people to do something we want them to do, make them active participants in doing something they want to do. Move from telling them to involving them. Using the word "You" a lot promotes greater patient involvement and patient-centered care. It gives people a sense of control over their decisions and outcomes.

The goal of imparting a sense of involvement and shared responsibility is so patients will be more committed to the process. As a rule, people tend to be more committed to their own ideas. Research has even demonstrated that when patients are involved in their care, they are more likely to remain compliant with treatment plans.[17]

No involvement. No commitment.

THE POWER OF COMMITMENT

Nobody likes to lose things! That's a point we made in the last chapter when discussing people's fear of loss. On that topic, I think it's safe to say most businesses would not want to lose $900,000 a year, but that's precisely what one Chicago restaurant was losing every year as a result of no-shows. Gordon's, a popular Chicago restaurant owned by Gordon Sinclair, found itself looking for ways to reduce its 30 percent no-show rate. Using a psychological approach, the restaurant was able to do this by making one simple change to the reservation process. In the past, when taking a reservation, a Gordon's employee would say, "Please call us if you change your plans." With this approach, three out of every ten reservations resulted in a no-show. However, once the statement was changed to a question that inspired a commitment, "Will you call us if you change your plans?", no-shows plummeted to 10 percent! The subtle shift was the receptionist's request for (and pause for) the caller's promise.[26]

From a psychological standpoint, the subtle but powerful difference was the first approach only required the caller to listen, the second approach required the caller to commit.

In the best-selling book *Influence: The Psychology of Persuasion* by Dr. Robert Cialdini, he devotes an entire chapter to the topic of commitment. Dr. Cialdini offers numerous examples of how our commitments can drive our actions and beliefs. For example, one study found that people at a racetrack were more confident of their horse's chances of winning immediately after they placed their bets. Another study found that when people were asked and agreed to collect donations for the American Cancer Society, there was a 700 percent increase in volunteers when a representative of the American Cancer Society called a few days later to ask for neighborhood canvassing. In yet another study, people were considerably more likely to intervene during a theft (in this study a theft was staged after a beach dweller walked away from her blanket) when the person was asked to "watch my things" as opposed to being a casual observer. 19 of 20 people who were asked to watch the person's belongings responded to the theft as opposed to only 4 of 20 who were not asked. According to Cialdini, "Once we make a choice or take a stand, we will encounter personal and interpersonal pressures to behave consistently with that commitment."[27] In short, not being consistent with our commitments is perceived as a character weakness associated with dishonesty and unreliability. Since most people do not want to be perceived this way, there is a greater internal and social pressure to do what we say.

According to the Journal of Personality and Social Psychology, when a person makes a public commitment, the desire to be consistent is so strong that the person's belief in what they committed to strengthens. The psychological principle behind commitments is that people desire to be consistent with their commitments.

This is extremely common in politics. Have you noticed that regardless of political affiliation, many people are willing to overlook a number of indiscretions and questionable decisions by politicians when the politician is the one they voted for? Even amidst numerous scandals and improprieties, people are reluctant to publicly condemn or turn their back on their candidate of choice. After all, this is the candidate they committed to!

Back to our example of the head nodding patient. Someone can nod their head back and forth so often that someone could confuse them for a bobble head doll, but there's no skin in the game with a head nod. The head nodder might not even agree with what you're saying or see the same importance as you. Sometimes we just nod our heads to be friendly or avoid conflict. If we aren't on the same page with someone trying to get us to do something, we will not be committed to taking action. If you want a true commitment that inspires action, it requires more than just a head nod. In health care, this involves the patient not only being an active participant in decisions that affect his or her care, but also adopting a model of shared responsibility between patient and clinician.

A MATTER OF INTENT

Above I referenced the book *Influence* by Dr. Cialdini. This is one of the most famous and renown books on the topic of influence and persuasion. Dr. Cialdini presents the data and compelling findings behind years of research into the principles that move people to change behaviors.

It's important to note, as made very clear in that book, that these principles can also be used for deceitful and malicious purposes. In fact, a large part of Dr. Cialdini's book focused on ways to defend yourself against these principles when they are being used against you for manipulative purposes.

The difference is really a matter of intent. The reason we feel uncomfortable and "on-guard" against traditional salespeople is because we fear they will attempt to manipulate us to buy a product or take an action that mostly benefits them, likely with a commission or a sale. Even though healthcare professionals prefer not to use the word "sell," there are many branches of health care where goods and services are indeed sold. Not to mention the wide range of non-sales selling required of people tasked with caring for the health of others and wanting to be influential in getting patients to assume responsibility for their health.

Being influential can be an extremely important skill when your intent is aligned with helping others, not manipulating them. This could be someone in a leadership position who oversees a team of employees, a coach tasked with improving the athletic abilities of his players, or a doctor responsible for improving health outcomes for the patients she sees.

As mentioned in the beginning of the book, the term "selling" has many connotations and often gets a bad rap because people associate selling with manipulation. In all fairness, that reputation is somewhat earned when you consider the amount of selling that involves trying to get someone else to do something that mostly benefits the seller. That is manipulation, and it's the exact opposite of what this book is about!

I want healthcare professionals to be more influential with patients so they will have greater IMPACT with improving the health and lives of the very people they serve.

If we're on the same page with that, let's move forward with becoming more influential in getting patients to share responsibility and accountability for doing the things that will lead to better health, improved outcomes, and greater satisfaction with the level of care they receive.

SMALL COMMITMENTS

In the world of traditional sales, there is something called "the close." Ugh! That's the part where someone has been talking your ear off about something you don't particularly want or need, and here it comes.. they want your money!

- If you buy today, you'll save 20 percent!
- Get it now while supplies last!
- We accept cash or credit!

Of course, all along you were nodding your head up and down leaving the impression that you couldn't wait to pull out your credit card and make this purchase. Can we all make a pact right now to stop doing the head nod?

While a traditional sales transaction may be different than the interaction that takes place between a patient and clinician, there are similarities in how people receive the information we provide and how they use that information to process decisions.

In the world of sales, salespeople often wait until the end of their presentation to make the big close. This is horribly ineffective if the potential buyer is not committed to moving forward.

What are some things that could get in the way of a sale?

- Failure to see the relevance of a product or solution
- Skepticism over information provided
- Price objection
- Conflict with personal preferences or lifestyle
- Wanting a simpler or more convenient solution

All through the presentation, the listener nodded his head while all these silent objections accumulated.

How likely is it that this person will move forward with a purchase? Probably not very likely.

Let's look at this from a health care perspective. What are some of the things that could prevent a patient from "buying" into your ideas or professional recommendations?

- Failure to see the relevance of a product or solution
- Skepticism over information provided
- Price objection
- Conflict with personal preferences or lifestyle
- Wanting a simpler or more convenient solution

That looks a lot like the list above! Are you starting to see that whether or not you embrace the term "salesperson," if you are in the business of influencing people and changing behaviors, you absolutely have to "sell" people!

Part of that involves getting commitments and overcoming objections. We'll take a deeper dive into overcoming objections in a later chapter, but for now I'll mention the value of getting small commitments from patients throughout the exam encounter as opposed to waiting for the end to drop the big close on them.

Research has shown that getting a series of small commitments is often more effective in getting people to comply with recommendations than waiting until the end and asking the person to make one BIG commitment.[27]

Here are a few examples of verbiage that can be sprinkled into your conversations with patients.

- Do you agree with what I'm saying?
- Are you ok with what I'm suggesting?
- Are you open to trying this?

From a psychological standpoint, these small commitments have a cumulative effect and make it easier for people to agree to a larger commitment asked of them later. It gives people a sense of involvement and control over their decisions, as opposed to the feeling that someone else is controlling them.

Of course, because we asked good questions, showed concern, and uncovered the patient's true desire for gain and fear of loss, the commitments we are asking of patients are directly aligned with what's important to them. That's a huge digression from a typical interaction with a salesperson more concerned about his commission than our well-being.

Nevertheless, people can still object for all kinds of reasons. While they may be on board with much of what you are saying, that doesn't mean there won't be some obstacles in the road that need to be addressed. Maybe there are significant financial concerns? Maybe they read something online that contradicted the information you are providing? Maybe they are leaving tomorrow for vacation and can't wait seven days for their contact lens order to arrive?

Regardless of the objection, it's better to get the patient to verbalize it earlier than later to see if it's something that can be successfully addressed. Asking for small commitments throughout your interaction time with a patient allows the patient an opportunity to object.

Doctor: *Are you ok with what I'm suggesting?*

Patient: *Well, sort of, but...*

Ok, let's deal with that now and see if there's a solution. Often, an objection is not a "no," it's a "maybe." Perhaps the patient just needs more information. Maybe he can't afford the medication you are prescribing. Maybe she travels for work and can't commit to the treatment regimen you are recommending. Maybe the objection can be overcome, or maybe it requires you to explore alternative options.

In chapter 7 we'll dig deeper into the best ways to deal with objections. For now, just know that objections, whether silent or verbalized, are a huge obstacle in your ability to get patients to act on the information you provide.

Involving patients in decisions that affect their health and getting them to verbally commit to the care process is a giant leap forward in your ability to not just educate patients, but actually IMPACT outcomes and results.

Who's the doctor here?

Maybe a better question, "Who's the patient here?"

CHAPTER FIVE

No Time Like Showtime

*"Do what you do so well that they will want
to see it again and bring their friends."*
~ Walt Disney

I mentioned earlier that I'm a naturally curious person. That being the case, I suppose it's no surprise that I frequently ask successful practice and business owners to describe what they feel has made them successful.

The answers, especially in service-based industries like health care, tend to focus on providing great service and a great experience for the people they serve. I've heard this reply so many times I come to expect it, but there was one individual whose reply was a bit more memorable.

This was an optometrist I was referred to for the purpose of discussing some business matters. We met at his practice. I was immediately impressed with his office, staff, technology and overall business model. Upon concluding our meeting, I asked him the question, "What's the number one thing you would credit your success to?"

Without pausing, he pointed toward the front entrance and said, "See that door over there?"

"Yes," I replied.

"Every time someone walks through that door, it's showtime," he said.

He went on to tell me that his entire team treated patients as if they were entering Disney World. He didn't have roller coasters or cotton candy, although that would have been really cool, but he did strive to create a memorable and "sticky" experience for his patients. He knew if the experience exceeded expectations (like Disney), people would not only return, but likely refer others. It worked, and they did.

Showtime. That word stuck with me. It got me thinking about my own interactions with patients and the experience I was creating. How could I make the experience more memorable and remarkable for patients?

To be honest, the experience I was providing at that time was pretty unremarkable. Typical paperwork followed by a wait. Some pretesting by a technician, and then I walked into the exam room. A little small talk, a couple questions, then I launched into a barrage of tests, followed by a review of my findings (where I probably used too much clinical jargon) and a prescription if needed.

Next!

It wasn't quite the Disney experience, more like a county fair. It shows up, people attend, it goes away. Spend some time at Disney and you'll have lifelong memories. Spend some time at a county fair and you'll have indigestion and memories of things you wish you could unsee. Ok, I guess we were better than a county fair, but I still had the lingering question, "What kind of show are we putting on?"

There's a reason people continue coming back to Disney. Once you've pushed through the turnstile, you're on stage. You're a guest, employees are cast members, and you are part of a show that doesn't end until you exit the park. Disney is a master at engaging the senses. Smells, sights, tastes, excitement, thrills, and anticipations. Your 4-year old points, and suddenly you're in line for an $18 ice cream cone. It doesn't matter. In spite of hot weather, long lines, and outrageous prices, over 150 million people visit Disney parks every year.

I'm not suggesting you start looping "It's a Small World" into your waiting area, and if you start wearing Mickey Mouse ears while examining patients, that's on you!

What I am suggesting is to make a "show" out of the information you provide and the manner in which you deliver it. Make it memorable, so it gets people's attention and makes them want to take action.

In the first few chapters we focused on exploring the patient's needs and concerns and getting the patient more involved and committed to their care. Just like the 4-year old who points directly at what's important to him (ice cream), we need patients to point us to what's important to them (hopefully it's not overpriced ice cream). Once we know that, it's time to start presenting them with solutions to their problems.

In this chapter I'll discuss multiple ways to do this more impactfully. Consistent with the book, these methods are based on psychological principals that make your message more memorable and impactful. Studies have found that people forget much of what they hear within 24 hours of hearing it. Yet another problem when you rely on "information" alone to make your case.

Here are some ways to deliver information more impactfully, with less likelihood of being dismissed or forgotten.

- Keep it simple
- Use visuals
- Create Contrast
- Tell stories
- Demonstrate enthusiasm
- Be likeable

KEEP IT SIMPLE

Over the years as a practicing optometrist I saw many patients show up to the office holding a broken or shattered pair of glasses. Perhaps they were run over by a car, chewed up by the family dog, or simply so old they just fell apart on their own. Unfortunately, on one family vacation many years ago, I was the unlucky individual presenting with a pair of broken glasses in hand after my 4-year-old seriously overestimated the bendability of titanium.

I had a current prescription, so I headed to a nearby optical shop to purchase a new pair. I was greeted by a friendly optician who led me to the various frame boards. I would estimate there was close to 800 frames to choose from. Hoping for some guidance and direction, the optician basically looked in the direction of the frame boards, then looked back at me and said, "Well, let me know when you find something you like."

To be clear, at no point did I mention I was an opto-metrist. Here's the reason. While I had graduated from optometry school, passed my state and national boards, practiced for several years and could diagnose and treat a plethora of visual abnormities and eye diseases, there was one area I admit to being fairly ignorant about. Eye fashion!

I didn't mention my occupation to the optician because I didn't want her to think I didn't need help. So, as she was migrating away from me, I politely regained her attention and asked if she could help me with my decision.

What styles are popular right now?

What are your top sellers?

What style would look good on my face?

I didn't ask those questions directly but that's the type of information I was looking for. Instead, she simply pointed out the various brand names, mentioned one of the brands they carried was new, and told me everything to the right of the sunglass stand was ladies frames. Then she smiled and walked away to "help" another customer.

I still recall standing in the middle of that optical, staring at 800+ frames and thinking to myself, "So this is what it feels like." By that I meant, this is what it feels like to be overwhelmed by choices.

I realized that the one thing I wanted at that time was for someone to make the decision easy and simple. That's it!

Back to the rider and elephant theme, let's look at what's happening in the brain in the situation above.

The rider likes to analyze things. In fact, it often does this to its detriment by overanalyzing and overthinking. The logical side of the brain really does want to make sense of the world and the situations it is presented with. However, a shortcoming of the rider is that it doesn't have tremendous reserves of mental energy. In situations that call for a high level of thinking and analyzing, the rider burns through mental fuel very quickly. Therefore, our brain relies on feelings for many of our decisions. While this doesn't always lead to the most logical or rational choices, it is nonetheless a more efficient way of processing information and coming to decisions.

The elephant, on the other hand, is lazy. What the elephant wants is quick, risk-free decisions. The more complex and convoluted the process becomes, the more likely the elephant is to turn around and head in the opposite direction.

That's exactly what happened that day in the optical. Overwhelmed by all the choices, my rider spun its wheels for a bit trying on different frames, until eventually the elephant turned around and walked out the front door. I wore an old pair of glasses the rest of the vacation.

Here is another example, based on a real medical case, of a doctor faced with an increased number of treatment options available to a patient. Imagine taking your 67-year old grandfather who had chronic hip pain from arthritis to his doctor for a checkup. In the past, your grandfather had been given drugs to treat his pain, but they were ineffective, so the doctor was forced to consider a more drastic option: hip replacement surgery. Obviously, this is a much more invasive process and requires a long and painful recovery process.

An unexpected break came when the pharmacy uncovered one medication that hadn't been tried. Now the doctor faced a dilemma. Should he prescribe the untried medication, even though the other one hadn't worked, or refer your grandfather for surgery?

This dilemma was created by physician Donald Redelmeier and psychologist Eldar Shafir to study the way doctors make decisions. When doctors were presented with this case history, 47 percent of them chose to try the medication in hopes of avoiding surgery.

In a variation of the dilemma, another group of doctors were presented with almost the same scenario, except this time the pharmacy discovered two untried medications. While this news of suddenly having two non-surgical options as opposed to one should be a thrill to both you and your grandfather, only 28 percent of the doctors presented with this scenario opted to try either one.[6]

From a logical standpoint, this doesn't make sense. The doctors are acting as if the mere existence of another medication made surgery a preferable option, but what is really taking place here is decision paralysis. More options, even good ones, can hinder our ability to make any decision at all. Or in this case, retreat to the default plan.

As healthcare professionals we don't want to oversimplify the information we provide to the point of preventing patients from having a full understanding of their condition or treatment options, but it would serve us and our patients well to keep our message compact. Healthcare professionals, by nature, are fascinated by nuance and complexity. That's when the Curse of Knowledge kicks in, and we start to forget what it's like *not* to know what we know. Accuracy to the point of uselessness is a symptom of the Curse of Knowledge. Simplifying a message doesn't have to devolve into "oversimplifying," but taking into consideration that people can learn and remember only so much information at once, compactness is worth striving for.

Keep it simple, but not too simple.

VISUALS

Every medical professional is very familiar with the term "noncompliance." This can be a hypertensive patient who routinely forgets to take his medication, someone who recently had knee surgery and ignores her doctor's recommendation for extended bedrest, or a teenager like mine who can't seem to remember to wear the rubber bands for his braces.

In optometry, there is a fair amount of noncompliance with contact lens use. Most brands of contact lenses have a recommended wearing time. Unfortunately, many patients ignore that recommendation.

One such patient happened to be a good friend of mine. For three straight years he presented with a worsening condition of corneal neovascularization from overuse of contact lenses. Corneal neovascularization, or CNV, is the in-growth of new blood vessels into avascular corneal tissue as a result of oxygen deprivation. In my friend's case, this was a result of sleeping in his contact lenses and wearing them beyond the recommended wearing time.

Corneal tissue is avascular in nature and the presence of vascularization can interfere with corneal transparency and optimal vision. If this blood vessel encroachment continued, that could cause a variety of symptoms including tearing, light sensitivity, redness, scarring and decreased vision.

For three years, I explained all of this to my friend, to which he replied with a sincere "I'm sorry. I'll try harder!" At this point, I wasn't buying it.

Instead of belaboring the point with more information about the dangers of contact lens overuse, an approach that had so far been unsuccessful, I decided to try a different approach. While he was giving me his annual list of excuses for why he couldn't stick with the recommended wearing schedule, I turned to my computer and produced a picture of corneal neovascularization. Even to someone not familiar with what a healthy eye should look like, this picture was, well… "gross."

I'll never forget his reaction. Without having to say a word, he looked at the image and immediately looked away.

"What is that?" he said. "Is that what you've been talking about? That looks awful! Is that what my eye looks like?"

Two things happened in that moment. One, he was suddenly a believer! Not only did he now understand the significance of the condition, but he started complying with recommendations. The other thing that happened was I suddenly realized the power of using visuals to make a point.

As it turns out this was not just an anomaly with my contact-lens abusing friend. Much of our sensory cortex is devoted to vision. In fact, the part of our brain responsible for processing words is quite small relative to the part of the brain that interprets visual images. A large body of research confirms that visual cues help us to better interpret, retrieve and remember information.[28]

Doctors and healthcare professionals educate people, correct? Of course, and by nature of that we are teachers. As a teacher, we want our students (patients) to understand and remember the information we are providing. Countless studies have confirmed the power of visual imagery in learning. One example is a study that asked students to remember groups of three words, such as dog, bike, and street. Students who made the effort to make a visual association with the three words, such as imagining a dog riding a bike down the street, did significantly better at recalling the three words than the ones who merely tried to memorize the words.[28]

In my role as a consultant, I do a lot of public speaking. When I first started, I would use a lot of bullet points in my presentations. Public speaking will teach you a lot about other people and what gets their attention based on their reaction to what you are saying or presenting. I learned early on that information alone was not very engaging.

"This is important information! Why is that lady in the fourth row staring at her phone, and why are those two guys in back carrying on a conversation?" While important, people quickly zone out when subjected to information overload. In public speaking, this is referred to as "death by bullet point."

What I came to realize all by myself (actually a speaking coach told me to knock it off with all the bullet points) was that images like pictures and videos were much more engaging to the audience. You could literally see people look up from their phones and stop conversing with a neighbor to pay attention, the same way I got my friend's attention with a picture. If you ever see me speak, you'll see that most of my slides are pictures and images that complement the message. I want people to focus on what

I'm saying but remember the image I used to make my point. Visuals make your message more "sticky."

Anatomically, the optic nerve is connected to the part of the brain responsible for feelings and emotion. We've all seen advertisements for weight loss products. These ads will often include some text discussing the science behind the product, or perhaps information about the ingredients in the formula. While this may be important information, is it really what drives sales? Is it memorable? Is it "sticky?"

How many advertisements for weight loss products do you see that do not have a before and after picture? Or at least a picture of someone who is in great physical health? It's the visual image that gets people to *feel* something. The elephant is motivated by feelings, not logic. The information is important to the rider, but without a motivated elephant, the rider is likely to analyze (quite possibly overanalyze) the information but not act on it. Studies have found that much of the information that we read or hear, when not accompanied by a visual image, is forgotten within twenty-four hours.[29]

Words are abstract and more difficult for the brain to retain. Think of the brain like an image processor, with much of the sensory cortex devoted to vision, as opposed to a word processor. We use words to express our thoughts, but we think in pictures. Images are more tangible, and therefore easier to encode and retain as opposed to abstract concepts.

When you hear the word cat, do you think of the three letters c-a-t or do you picture a cat? Most likely, you called to mind an image of a cat. When you hear the word diabetes what do you see? Probably not much because abstract concepts are difficult to visualize and therefore harder to encode.

Think about it. How many patients return to you for a yearly exam and say, "I've been thinking about that 3rd side effect you mentioned at our last exam"? Yet that's how doctors often educate, using abstract concepts that fail to "stick" in the patient's memory.

This was the problem I had with my contact-lens abusing friend (I'll stop calling him that now – he does have a name). The information I was giving him was abstract. It sounded really important to me when I heard myself say it, but obviously didn't have the same impact on him. The picture, on the other hand, created a "feeling." It was memorable and gave my words new meaning. It got him to change!

Information is important, but it's also quickly forgotten. Whenever possible, supplement your verbal information with visuals. Visuals are memorable and easily retrieved. In the quest to be more influential and persuasive with patients, it would be wise to use a lot of visuals when making a case for behavior change.

CONTRAST

Another tool for making change simple for the patient while demonstrating value is contrast. Optometrists execute this as part of routine eye care, perhaps without even realizing it.

"Which is better, one or two?"

This is the classic question that optometrists ask their patients when doing a refraction to find the patient's eyeglass prescription. Sometimes we get crazy and use letters instead of numbers!

If you're an optometrist reading this, you can certainly identify with the following. Patients love when the choice is obvious. They are very comfortable and confident with their replies.

Doctor: *Which is better, one or two?*

Patient: *One is better!*

Doctor: *How about now?*

Patient: *This time number two is better! Hey, this is fun. I'm acing this test! I'll probably have super-human vision!*

When does this test start to become not so fun for the patient? It's when the choices become difficult.

Doctor: *Ok, how about now?*

Patient: *[Long pause]. I'm not sure doc. They look about the same. Can I see them again? [Another long pause]. I'm still not sure. I'm afraid to pick one. What if I make a bad choice and get the wrong prescription?*

At this point the once very confident patient suddenly becomes noncommittal and indecisive.

If you're not in the eye care field and you've felt this way before as a patient getting an eye examination, please take comfort that this point of indecisiveness is exactly where we are trying to get you. When you're at a point where the choices look similar and it's very difficult to decide, that's how we know we have the correct prescription dialed in.

For the sake of a refraction, this is good. Indecisive and non-committal is exactly where we need you. But it's really bad for sales, whether that's selling a pair of glasses or "selling" a patient on why they need to eat healthier.

There is some overlap in these categories and I already eluded to an example of contrast in the visuals section above. A weight loss advertisement is a great example. The before and after picture! The advertisers are hoping that people who see the ad will identify with the before picture but be motivated to want to look like the after picture. It's a powerful combination of visuals and contrast.

We've discussed that it's the emotional side of our brain that often motivates us to act. The emotional side of our brains cannot analyze things nearly as well as the logical side of our brain. The emotional side struggles with the concept of past and future. It's very present minded. That being the case, it struggles to comprehend words or descriptions of past or future.

When it's possible to demonstrate contrast, take advantage of that. Don't just tell me how much my health will improve if I change a behavior, show me. The emotional side of the brain is sensitive to solid contrast such as before/after, risky/safe, with/without, and slow/fast.

Contrast allows the decision-making part of the brain to make quick, risk-free decisions without a lot of analyzing and contemplation. It's not that we don't want patients to contemplate decisions that impact their health, but we want to avoid a cycle of overanalyzing that leads to no decision at all. Without contrast, the old brain enters a state of confusion, which ultimately results in delaying a decision or worse yet, avoiding a decision altogether.

When the brain sees competing options, it will assess each and select the best. Many studies in consumer behavior have found that when people are given one item to choose from, they lack confidence to make a decision. When two options are presented, the perception of risk and fear is lessened, and the consumer is more confident in making a decision.

As consumers, we find ourselves frequently assessing the pros and cons of making one decision or purchase over another. In health care, a similar process takes place when presented with competing options involving our health and lifestyle. As discussed throughout this book, often the option is to change or not to change.

Whether you sell a product, a service, or you're simply trying to "sell" patients on the benefits of taking a certain action or changing a behavior, amplify your message by demonstrating contrast whenever possible. Highlight what sets your practice and brand apart with a stark comparison between your product and the competition or how life is now and how it would be without following your advice.

Which is better, one or two?

Make the choice obvious!

FACTS TELL. STORIES SELL.

Imagine having one minute to make a persuasive pitch to someone. With only sixty seconds to work with, you decide to mention a few facts in your effort to persuade someone to do what you are asking them to do. Since the focus of this book is health care, let's assume you are attempting to persuade an overweight patient to start exercising. Let's further assume you took this approach with one hundred patients over the course of a month. Below are the 3 facts you chose to share.

- People who are physically active for approximately seven hours a week are 40% less likely of dying early than people who are only active for less than 30 minutes a week.
- Only 10% of people are successful at losing weight through diet alone.
- Even 10 minutes of exercise will help raise your heart rate and maintain fitness levels.

What you weren't aware of is that all these patients were accompanied to the exam by a family member who waited patiently in the waiting area while you examined the patient. On the ride home, the family member asked, "So, what did the doctor tell you?" Would you be surprised to discover that only 5 percent of these one hundred patients could recall the statistics you shared?

Instead of sharing statistics about fitness and exercise, let's assume you chose to share a story about a patient of yours who refused to exercise and was now being treated by you for multiple health complications. Or perhaps you shared a story about a patient with similar medical conditions who transformed his health and quality of life by simply walking outdoors for thirty minutes every morning, able to slowly wean off his medications and now enjoying a much fuller and more active life. Would these stories be more memorable than statistics?

In one study researchers asked students to make a one-minute persuasive pitch to other members in their class. On average, students used 2.5 statistics in their pitch. Only 1 in 10 told a story. Ten minutes later, researchers asked everyone to pull out a piece of paper and write down every single idea they could remember. Only 5% remembered any statistic. 63% of the students remembered the story.[30]

Stories are memorable in ways that statistics are not. When statistics are presented, certain parts of the brain are activated – Broca's and Wernicke's Area. These areas are specialized for comprehension of human language. When these parts of the brain are activated, we can understand but we cannot feel. When a story is shared, it stirs up an emotion. Our whole brain is activated. Greater meaning is extracted when people can relate to the story and feel a personal connection.

Our brains are not hardwired to retain facts for very long. Our brains are hardwired to retain stories. When data and stories are shared together, the listener is moved both intellectually and emotionally.

Stories move people to take action. A focus of this book is on getting people to "feel" something on an emotional level that prompts them to act. Think about what you want the person to do, feel or think after hearing a story. The more emotionally invested we are in something, the more motivated we are to change.

Stories breathe life into the benefits of change in ways that facts and statistics don't. Stories are relatable and powerful. Through this connection, the patient realizes this isn't just something that happens to other people, this has happened to people you see and could also happen to me!

Beyond "feeling" something, stories literally change our brain chemistry. Certain chemicals are released in the body when we hear a story. Communication and storytelling expert David JP Phillips refers to the following three chemicals as the "angel's cocktail." These are dopamine, oxytocin and endorphins.[31]

Dopamine increases focus, motivation and memory. All stories are dopamine creating. When we are presented with a story, such as when we read a book, we create situations in our mind around this scenario. We imagine the characters and the environment. The story becomes vivid and memorable in our mind in a way that facts and statistics do not.

Endorphins boost happiness. When we watch a funny movie, endorphins cause us to laugh. Endorphins cause people to become more focused, creative and relaxed. High levels of endorphins, such as during rigorous exercise, can even lead to a feeling of euphoria.

Oxytocin has the effect of making people more generous. People will trust you more and will become more likely to bond with you. In storytelling, you create empathy. Oxytocin is one of the most beautiful chemicals of all, because it makes us feel human.

Stories literally change behavior by changing brain chemistry!

Contrast the effect of these chemicals with what David JP Phillips refers to as the "devil's cocktail." These are cortisol and adrenaline. In high concentrations, these chemicals cause people to become intolerant, irritable, uncreative, critical, memory impaired, and often lead to bad decisions.

If your goal is to create a psychological state that increases the chances that someone will move in a direction you want them to, what state do you think is more conducive to this?

Stories make us feel something, and as we've demonstrated, many of our decisions are determined by feelings, not logic. You don't have to become a master storyteller, just start collecting stories and share with patients when appropriate. This will make you much more interesting to patients, while also enhancing your ability to get their attention and deliver a more memorable and impactful message.

Ever wonder why almost every Ted Talk is a story and not a regurgitation of facts and data delivered by bullet-point? Well, now you know.

ENTHUSIASM SELLS

One of my first jobs in the optometric profession was working at a retail optical as a doctor's technician. I believe I started this job during my first year of optometry school. At this early stage of my education, I didn't have a deep wealth of knowledge on eye care, but as they say, "I knew enough to be dangerous."

As an incentive bonus, the company I worked for offered what they called "spiffs." These were essentially bonuses based on production and paid out quarterly. The intent, as with many production bonuses, was to motivate employees to perform at a higher level. Similar to what healthcare professionals want patients to do regarding changing something that will improve their health or well-being, the company wanted the employees to *change* their approach to patient care in ways that would drive greater revenues. The assumption was if we incentivize employees with money, they will become more motivated and enthused to produce at a higher level. In reality, I didn't see much change in employee behavior by having this spiff. It was just an extra check we received once a quarter.

After a few months working at this position while concurrently attending optometry school, we began learning about an eye condition called presbyopia. Presbyopia happens when the eye's natural lenses become less flexible. This inhibits the eye's natural ability to focus. For many patients, one of the first signs is having to hold reading materials further and further away to read clearly. This usually happens somewhere after hitting the big 4-0. Patients will often joke that their arms are getting shorter.

One day, while going through my typical routine of working up a patient prior to seeing the doctor, the 40-something patient in front of me mentioned that it has become much more difficult to focus at near. I handed him a near point card (eye chart to assess visual acuity at reading distance) and he could only read the larger size letters. He was pulling the card away to see it clearer. For many people, this would be a mundane observation. As a first-year optometry student, I lit up like a Christmas tree!

Enthusiasm is the X Factor when it comes to selling, but where does it come from? I believe that enthusiasm can be developed by combining three simple elements. Looking back, these are the same three things that contributed to my enthusiasm treating the patient in the example above.

1. Curiosity. In the world of sales, great salespeople enjoy probing into a client's problem. Great salespeople are not enthusiastic because they solved a

problem, they solve a problem because they are enthusiastic. This starts with questions and curiosity. When the patient above indicated that he was having difficulty reading at near, I launched into a series of questions to learn more about this problem. Knowing that I had the knowledge to help this person (discussed below), enthusiasm picked up speed with every answer.

2. Knowledge. If a topic is of little interest to you, you will have no desire to be enthusiastic. But when you do learn something new, you begin to understand its importance and your enthusiasm accelerates. The more you know, the more enthusiastic you become because you can see more opportunities and provide more insights to people who will benefit from your knowledge. While most healthcare professionals have a high level of knowledge in their respective fields, only a minority become "gurus" in some area of their specialty. These are often the ones who write and speak on their area of expertise and gain local or even national notoriety for their expert status. They love sharing what they know, and their enthusiasm is infectious.

3. Belief. With a better understanding of the patient's problems and armed with knowledge that could help this poor patient who was struggling to read, I became enthusiastic with the belief that I could help him. I wasn't thinking about a spiff or anything that

involved personal gain, I was solely focused on how I could share my knowledge and expertise to help him resolve his problem. Maybe some people are better actors than me, but I wasn't able to fake enthusiasm to get a higher spiff. You must believe what you are saying. When you have a high level of knowledge about a topic and truly believe you can help someone, you can't help but enthusiastically share that information. Genuine enthusiasm is intrinsic – it comes from within.

Whether you are attempting to sell a pair of glasses or sell someone on why they need to eat healthier or start exercising, enthusiasm sells. The best thing you can do is maintain focus on the other person's problems and how you can help that person. When the focus shifts to "upselling" to create more revenue for the practice or a one-size-fits-all approach to selling that mostly benefits the practice's bottom line, you can expect that your enthusiasm and the enthusiasm of those on your team will decline. You might be excited at the prospect of making more money, but efforts to get the patient to follow your recommendations will not feel or come across as genuine. If you or your employees are not enthusiastic about all the ways you can help someone, you can expect the patient to not be enthused about what you are recommending.

Conversely, if you are enthused, that emotional state can be transferred to the other person. This is called emotional contagion. A massive experiment of almost 700,000 people showed that emotional states can be transferred to others, leading people to experience the same emotions without their awareness. Emotional contagion is also well established in controlled studies, with people transferring positive and negative emotions to others.[32]

Develop a high level of curiosity about your patients. Become a guru while others in your field (even doctors) continue to operate as generalists. Most importantly, believe with full conviction in what you are telling someone.

As medical professionals, we typically try to avoid exposing people to things that are contagious. Enthusiasm is an exception.

LIKEABILITY

I've had the privilege of visiting many optometry practices for the purpose of observing. As a practice management consultant, I'm constantly observing successful practice owners and looking for commonalities. I've adopted this practice in many areas of my own life. When I meet someone who is financially successful, I strike up a conversation about what they do for a living. When I'm at the gym, I look for the most physically fit people and pay attention to their workout routine. Studying high performers and adopting their habits can accelerate your path to success.

If you pay close enough attention, you sometimes recognize the not-so-obvious qualities that make someone successful. Over time, I started to recognize a certain pattern with successful practice owners. They were genuinely likeable!

When the doctor would walk into the room, the patient would immediately smile. This wasn't a reaction intended to simply conform to social norms of being friendly and polite, it was a smile that communicated the patient was genuinely happy to see their doctor.

Hey! How are you doing? Great to see you! How are the kids?

There was an immediate connection. There was a spirit of friendliness in the air. I watched the doctor interact with the patient, giving full attention to their every word. There was eye contact, positive body language, smiling, laughing, and compassion. The patient was leaning in, not away. There was a high level of trust, respect and likeability communicated in their mannerisms.

It's difficult to quantify the impact of likeability as it relates to the success of these practices, but I got the impression from these interactions that the patient was more likely to be on board with the doctor's recommendations and less likely to seek products and services from other sources.

What makes people like (and dislike) their doctors? That's a question asked by a company called Zocdoc, a platform for medical appointments and patient feedback. Zocdoc culled their database of reviews to determine what factors mattered most in positive and negative reviews of healthcare providers. Perhaps not surprisingly, the most common word used in positive reviews was "friendly."[33]

While it's probably no surprise that people prefer their doctors and healthcare professionals to be friendly, let's consider what role this plays in a doctor's ability to be influential with people.

There is a saying that goes, "people do business with people they know, like, and trust." Each one of these qualities influences the others. We tend to place higher levels of trust in people or companies that we like. The next chapter is devoted to establishing trust with people. Research has also shown that familiarity with a company or brand promotes likeability, unless the experience was bad.

There is an idea in social psychology called the *mere exposure effect*. Numerous studies have found that the more times people are exposed to a person, brand or company, the more they like that person, brand or company! This "mere exposure" also makes people more likely to say yes to someone whom they are familiar with and like, as opposed to someone they feel neutral toward.

In a Stanford study, MBA students at Stanford and Northwestern were put into negotiation situations. Students were randomly assigned partners and given the same deal to negotiate. The only difference was that one group was instructed to focus strictly on business, while the other group was asked to get to know their partner through email exchanges, sharing photos, and things like that. The group that kept it strictly business was 5 times more likely to fail in the negotiation because they didn't come to like the other person. It was easier to say no.

It's important to consider that the people in the all business group probably didn't dislike each other, but they were relatively neutral toward one another. I think in most cases this more accurately describes doctor and patient interactions. Neutrality is not the same as genuine likeability. In the same way people don't recommend an average restaurant or an average movie, they also don't recommend a doctor who provided an "average" experience.

When we genuinely like someone, we experience positive emotions. Scientific studies have found that when we are in a positive emotional state, we have increased comprehension and enhanced mental capacity to make decisions and increased receptiveness to persuasive requests. When we are in a negative emotional state, the result is clouded judgment and difficulty seeing value in what is being presented.

Above we discussed emotional contagion. This is a not so hidden secret of great customer service in the retail world.

When you improve the emotional state of shoppers, they will be more predisposed to do business with you. I believe this receptiveness can be applied to health care as well.

Below are a few ways to be more likeable in the eyes of your patients:

- Like your patients! Find something you like about the patient and mention it. We tend to like people who like us.
- Discuss topics this stimulate good feelings, such as kids, hobbies or vacations.
- Make notes in the patient's chart about personal interests and inquire about this at future visits.
- Smile often. It's hard to remain in a foul mood when someone keeps smiling at you.
- Use humor. Humor has actually been identified as one of the qualities that makes doctors less likely to be sued![34]
- Familiarity. Discussed above. Get involved in your community. Create awareness for your practice and brand through marketing. Join clubs or groups where you can meet new people.
- Be relatable. Find common interests. Who says you can't talk about cooking or music at a medical exam?
- Avoid the mood killers! Reduce or eliminate long waits, inconveniences and rude service. Your practice is a reflection on you.

IT'S SHOWTIME

This chapter was titled "No Time Like Showtime" because I wanted to highlight the importance of creating an environment and experience where people would be moved to change something based on your recommendations.

Think about how you "show up" for your patients. Don't dilute your message to the point of oversimplification, but do keep it simple. Use visuals whenever possible to supplement your verbal information. Make choices easier by demonstrating contrast when presenting options. Allow empathy (desire to help the patient) and authority (possessing the knowledge and expertise to solve their problem) drive your enthusiasm, a feeling that will be transferred to the other person. And for Pete's sake, be likeable!

Now get out there and break a leg!

CHAPTER SIX:

Earn Trust

"How do you develop trust? It's simple: you show your genuine sense of concern for their well-being. Then trust will come."
~ The Dalai Lama

I'm going to start off this chapter with a hard truth. Your patients don't trust you.

Before you defiantly dismiss that assertion, let's unpack that comment and take a closer look.

There was a time when a lab coat and a medical degree garnered immediate and complete trust. Doctors were authority figures who commanded people's attention. Because the level of trust was so high, a doctor's ability to influence others was high as well. The advice and recommendations of doctors had a strong influence over patient's decisions and overall health outcomes. They didn't have to *sell* patients on change, patients just did what their doctor recommended. Doctor knows best!

We live in a different time. While healthcare professionals are still revered for their knowledge and generally respected in the eyes of their community, we must acknowledge that the level of trust placed in doctors and the healthcare institution in general has declined over the years.

We have learned in our exploration of trust that there are multiple drivers of low trust in the medical field. Competing and contradictory sources of information have become prevalent. Patients needing medical procedures seek out multiple opinions from doctors, which can only be assumed to imply a lack of trust. Every day, through social media and a variety of other outlets, we read about miracle cures that have no basis in scientific fact. A recent Google search for "popular fake medical news" delivered a staggering 240 million results. Conflicts of interest and lack of disclosure are also factors impacting trust.

There are additional challenges with healthcare practices that sell products or services. If you still don't like the word "sell," then fine! Use "prescribe" or whatever word you're comfortable with. From the patient's perspective, it doesn't matter what you call it, it only matters how they perceive it. For an optometrist, every patient walking into your optical thinks you sell glasses. Same with a dentist selling teeth whitening kits or a chiropractor selling heating pads for sore muscles. Consumers are innately distrustful of people attempting to sell them something. Even healthcare professionals are not immune to that.

In 1975, 80% of the public had confidence in the medical system. Contrast that with a Gallup poll conducted in 2018 that found only 34% of the general public had a positive view of the healthcare industry.[35]

I repeat, your patients do not trust you.

To put a positive spin on this, let me rephrase that statement. Your patients don't trust you YET. And obviously I'm not talking about all your patients. Certainly, if you've been in practice for a while you've earned the trust of many of your patients. However, to my earlier point, it probably wasn't your lab coat and degree that got the job done. This is an area that many healthcare professionals struggle to accept.

But I'm a doctor, damnit!

Yes, you are, and a lot of people don't give a damn about your title! Educate all you want, but patients continue to not exercise, not floss daily, not return for regular exams, and not take their contact lenses out at night. If everyone followed your advice you wouldn't be yelling, "But I'm a doctor, damnit!"

What's my point? I'm glad you asked. My point is that we need to shed the ego and be more proactive in building trust with our patients and the people in our community. Trust is so important! It directly correlates with our ability to be influential. Without influence, it's hard to get people to change.

So, here's what I want you to do. Burn the lab coat and throw your degree in the garbage!

Ok, you don't really have to do that. It's more of a symbolic request.

What I would like you to do is look beyond your title and focus on the things that really build trust in the eyes of your patients. In essence, this entire book is about building trust, but in this chapter I want to focus on three key areas that drive trust for healthcare professionals. As you read along, you may feel that you are already integrating these things into your practice and professional brand, but I'll ask you to consider if you could be doing more to build trust.

We know from peer-reviewed research that patients who have more trust in their healthcare professionals are more satisfied with their treatment, have fewer symptoms and pursue healthier behaviors.[36] Considering this book is about influencing change, pay special attention to that last one – pursue healthier behaviors! Education without action is useless. Getting patients to change behaviors is magical.

Let's get into the three areas. They are Authority, Capabilities and Results.

AUTHORITY

While you are struggling with getting your patients to follow simple instructions such as lose weight, wear sunglasses outdoors, or return for an annual exam, imagine having so much influence with people that you were able to coerce someone into delivering electric shocks to another person when that person failed at a task.

Did that get your attention?

In 1974, an experiment was conducted by a psychology professor named Stanley Milgram to study how punishment affects learning and memory. One participant in the study, referred to as the Learner, had the task of learning pairs of words in a long list until each pair could be recalled perfectly. The other participant's job was to deliver increasingly strong electric shocks for every mistake. This person was called the Teacher.

You might assume the Teacher, having not been aware of his role in this experiment until he showed up at the laboratory suite, would refuse to continue with the experiment as the voltage levels increased to dangerous levels. However, many of the participants in the Teacher role were willing to deliver continued, intense, and dangerous levels of shock to a kicking, screeching, pleading Learner.

In fact, about two-thirds of the subjects pulled every one of the thirty shock switches in front of them, from 195 volts all the way to 450 volts until the researcher ended the experiment. More alarming, almost none of the 40 subjects quit his job as Teacher when the victims first began to demand, even beg, for his release.[27]

This is unsettling to the point of being nightmarish! There's only one caveat I failed to mention. No real shock was ever delivered. The Learner was an actor who only pretended to be in agony. The actual purpose of the study was to determine how much suffering ordinary people would be willing to inflict on an entirely innocent person.

This experiment begs the question, "What could make people do such things?" Follow-up studies ruled out factors such as gender, age, and psychological states of the subjects. As it turned out, the predominant influence in this case was determined to be a deep-seated sense of duty to authority. According to Milgram, the subjects were unable to defy the wishes of the boss, the lab-coated researcher who directed the subjects to perform their duties.

While the ethical standards of this experiment may be questionable, it does demonstrate an impressively high level of authority demonstrated by a healthcare professional, although keep in mind this experiment was conducted in 1974. Here is a question I would like you to ponder.

In today's healthcare environment, do doctors and medical professionals still have a high level of authority with patients?

I think the answer is yes, but I also think that authority has declined over the years. From the standpoint of having influence over the patients we treat, I think we've lost some of that. It's one of the reasons I wrote this book.

Patients now have access to information. Dr. Google is a legitimate competitor of ours. The information medical professionals provide is no longer exclusively accessible through a doctor. There are numerous channels popping up for receiving healthcare products and services outside the care of a licensed physician.

While there are pros and cons to having healthcare information widely available, I do believe it has chipped away at the perception people have of healthcare providers. The ability to quickly go online and search symptoms and treatments and in many cases order healthcare products and services without ever having to interact with a doctor has changed the landscape of medicine and the perception of healthcare providers. The bottom line is that the public does not need us as much as they used to, and that has slowly eroded our social influence.

Please understand I'm fully aware of the pitfalls of self-diagnosis and treatment, but I'm coming at this from a public perception angle, and perception becomes reality for people! So, how do we change that perception?

The way you change it is to reclaim your authority! I'm sorry, but a lab coat and a degree does not carry the weight that it used to. It's a good start, but let me challenge you to take it to the next level.

One of my son's baseball coaches arranged for the team to be evaluated by, in the coach's words, the "best" physical therapist in the state of Georgia. Wow! That's quite a title. The physical therapist was going to assess the players strengths and weaknesses as it related to all their joints and their range of motion. Feedback would be provided, and corrective actions would be prescribed to avoid injuries during the season. And all of this would be provided by the BEST physical therapist in the entire state!

Then I thought, "Wait a minute, how does someone get to be the best at this?" It's not like a sporting event where there's a clearly defined winner. Was there a contest that determined this? Was there a test that PTs could take that resulted in a ranking system? Was there somebody who had the job of visiting every physical therapist in the entire state and then deciding on who was the best?

Here's the thing about being the best at something. It's often based on perception. Let's imagine you visited two different eye care physicians for chronic dry eyes. The first physician treated your condition but gave no indication that he or she had superior knowledge or competencies relative to other physicians. You probably would have gotten the sense that you could have gone to any eye care physician and received similar treatment. Now let's contrast this with the second practitioner. When you walk into her office, you see advanced degrees on the wall for specialized dry eye certifications. Next to the certifications are framed articles the doctor has published on innovative treatments for dry eye conditions. As you take a seat in the waiting area, you realize one of the reading selections is a self-published book on dry eye written by the doctor, and a video is running overhead of the doctor being interviewed for a local news broadcast on the increasing prevalence of dry eye with increased digital device usage.

Given the two options, who would you place more trust in? Who would you be more likely to say was the *best* dry eye doctor in your area? Who would you be more likely to refer a friend to who complained about having dry eyes?

In the world of heath care, competency does matter. You can't claim to be the best and then not deliver on that. In the business world, this happens frequently. Companies invest in slick, persuasive marketing campaigns claiming their product or service is superior to the competition, but the actual product or service doesn't live up to that claim. A restaurant can claim they have the best food and service, but when you show up and the restaurant is not clean, nobody brings you water, the waitress is rude, and your medium rare steak shows up well done, any gains the restaurant attained from their "story" about being the best will likely be short-lived. So, whether you're a doctor, restaurant owner, or sell T-shirts on the side of the road, you must deliver on your claims.

While competency matters, so does perception. When I lived in Chicago, there was an Irish bar near my apartment that claimed to sell the 5th best hamburger in the city. In a small town, the 5th best anything might not be an impressive claim, but in a city the size of Chicago, the 5th best burger is pretty impressive!

Ironically, this particular Irish bar never made one single hamburger. In fact, they didn't even have a kitchen. What they did have was a back door, and if you opened that back door and walked across an alley, you would come to the back entrance of a steak restaurant that was voted to have the 5th best hamburger in the city of Chicago. The Irish bar contracted with the steak restaurant to provide their food. They didn't make hamburgers, but in the mind of their customers they offered one of the best burgers in the city!

This isn't exactly an apples to apples comparison because doctors and healthcare providers usually do provide the products and services they offer, but I use that example to highlight perception. To use our dry eye example, it's possible both doctors were equally knowledgeable and qualified to treat your dry eye. It's even possible the first doctor was more qualified, but you made a determination on who was more qualified based more on perception than actual competencies.

People rarely if ever ask their healthcare providers where they attended school or where they ranked in their class.

In no way am I minimizing the value of education, advanced training and medical competency in treating patients, but with the focus of this book on getting people to change, let's not overlook perception. If you are a very qualified physician but people perceive you as just another option on a long list of providers, you will have less influence with your patients than a practitioner who people perceive to be the best, or at least in the category of "the best."

CAPABILITIES

It's true that perception is reality, but reality is also reality, and reality can quickly change one's perception.

In the section on authority, I wanted to highlight the value of perception and branding and how that factors into the level of trust people place in you. However, if you want to be known as the "best" in a particular area, it has to involve more than just perception. You must deliver on capabilities.

Speaking from the position of an optometrist, we get excellent training in optometry school. Our training and education allow us to provide a wide scope of care for both visual abnormalities and ocular disease. Despite a stellar educational program, most practice owners hiring recent optometry school graduates express concern with this, suggesting it will take some time for the young doctor to get "up to speed."

This is a fair concern. When I first started practicing, even patients would sometimes call my age into question. Many of us have a fear that when a young (or young looking) doctor steps into the room he or she will lack the experience needed to provide competent care. I recall one particularly outspoken patient of mine that looked me straight in the eye about five minutes into the exam and said, "Are you old enough to be a doctor?" At the time I recall being offended by that question. Years later, when they stop asking, that's when you start to miss it! For the record, if anyone wants to "offend" me by pointing out how young I look, I won't hold it against you!

But I digress. My point is to continue developing your competencies as a clinician. Obviously, this will happen passively as you see more patients and gain more experience. I recall a doctor I interned for telling me that 90 percent of the ocular abnormalities I referred to a specialist during my first year in practice would be conditions I would be comfortable treating or monitoring myself by my second year in practice. He was right. With experience came more confidence, and confidence breeds trust.

Healthcare professionals are also required to complete a certain number of continuing education hours as a requirement to renew their license. And I'm sure you regularly read articles, periodicals or other resources to stay current with your clinical abilities. So, you're developing your knowledge and capabilities. I get it. But that doesn't necessarily make you an "expert" in the minds of patients. You're just doing what every other professional in your position is doing. As discussed, that may not be enough to reinforce a high level of trust with patients and prospective patients. I'll challenge you to kick it up a notch or three.

To the example of the "best" physical therapist in Georgia, I decided to visit his website to learn more about him. His accolades were lengthy and impressive. I had been to physical therapists in the past and while I respected their craft, I admit to having a "one size fits all" perception of the therapists I had seen. I trusted them to the point that they knew more than I did, but still wondered if the therapy I was receiving was the best option. Would a different therapist give different advice or offer a different treatment regimen? Should I even be going to a physical therapist? Why not a chiropractor or a massage therapist?

This doesn't sound like a high level of trust, does it? As a patient, you've probably found yourself in a similar scenario at times. As a clinician, patients have likely felt this way about you at times.

But I didn't have these reservations or concerns with this particular physical therapist, and it was due in large part to authority and capabilities. Based on the coach's comments, I adopted the perception (often times we base our perceptions on other people's perceptions) that this particular physical therapist provided elite care, maybe even the "best" in the area, and he had the credentials to validate that.

Unless you're continually improving your skills, you're quickly becoming irrelevant. And when you're irrelevant, you're no longer credible. And without credibility, trust diminishes.

In eye care, there are numerous options for getting advanced training, degrees and certifications for various specialties. I'm sure those options exist for most medical professions. Find an area that particularly interests you and grow your competencies in that area. Invest in your education. Develop your skills. Train under other experts if you have the opportunity. Seek out programs that offer certifications. Invest in the technology to provide care at a level your competitors can't. You don't have to be the best at everything, but find niches within your field that you're passionate about and become the best at that. Remember, the "best" is a subjective term that's often based on perception, but it's also based on your capabilities. Work to develop both.

Becoming the foremost expert in your area of influence is the single most important thing you can do to build your brand and establish trust. When people ask, "Who's the best person around for treating XYZ condition," be the one they name.

What they're really asking is, "Who can I *trust* with my health?"

RESULTS

I saved the greatest trust building key for last. Results!

This is the beauty of following the advice in this book. You may have chosen to read this book because you weren't getting the results you wanted. If you're a chiropractor, patients weren't doing their at-home stretches between sessions. If you're a sports medicine physician, patents weren't compliant with their rehab exercises. If you're an optician, patients weren't "buying into" your recommmendations to purchase multiple pairs of glasses for various uses.

I've heard this repeatedly in the eye care profession and I've heard a similar sentiment from medical professionals of other specialties. "Patients don't follow our advice!" Of course, this doesn't apply to all patients, but if a large segment of your patient base is opting to forego your professional recommendations, this will negatively impact the results you create in your practice.

Let's contrast this with a doctor or practice that routinely creates results for the patients they serve. In other words, more patients are "sold" on the cure they are offered. This practice will produce more results! Consistently producing results for patients not only causes patients to return, it also compels them to consistently recommend you to others.

Think about it. When someone needs a medical procedure done, they often inquire, "Who's the best doctor to see for this?" You don't want to see just *any* cardiologist, or periodontist, or ophthalmologist. You want assurance that the person you see is highly competent. Both capabilities and results are matters of competence. We trust people who are highly capable and make good things happen. These people have influence. Without influence, you end up doing a lot of talking to people who don't take action. When you have influence, you have the ability to get people to take action. The result of action is results!

I won't pretend to be an expert on all medical specialties, so I'll use eye care as the example here. There are several areas within eye care that an optometrist can specialize. The same can be said for ophthalmologists and opticians (we call these the 3 O's in the industry). In optometry, you can specialize in dry eye treatment. You can become a pediatric expert specializing in children with vision disorders like strabismus and convergence insufficiency. You can be a sports vision specialist focused on helping athletes with vision-related issues like peripheral awareness and tracking skills. Whatever your specialty, it's ultimately results that will be the biggest driver of trust.

Are your dry eye patients now your raving fans because they no longer have to peel their contact lenses out of their eyes after a long day of staring at a computer?

Are your athlete patients reporting back to you how much better they are performing on the playing field since starting treatment with you?

Have a few moms cried because their child can now read and do homework without seeing double vision?

If so, then you're getting results! Whatever healthcare profession you are in, are you getting impressive results? Not just the kind of results people expect you to get (everyone *expects* an optometrist to prescribe an accurate glasses prescription), but the kind of results that make people say, "Wow!"

If you've ever watched the television show *Shark Tank*, you've likely seen the "sharks," the panel of wealthy investors who listen to presentations delivered by aspiring entre-preneurs, offer their candid impressions of the presenter's product. The sharks are quick to condemn a product and not bashful with their candid first impressions. Kevin O'Leary, also known as "Mr. Wonderful" on the show, is fond of the term "poo-poo on a stick" when referring to products and inventions he doesn't like.

But no matter how bad the first impression, there's one thing that quickly changes their minds. Results! Initially, the inventor makes a lot of claims about the product and its market potential. Inevitably, the presenter is asked about sales. Sometimes the sales number confirm the shark's impression that the product is indeed poo-poo on a stick. However, there are times when the sales are extremely impressive. An amazing thing happens at this point. Every shark sits up a little straighter in his or her chair and takes notice. They go from ridiculing the product to seeking a business partnership with the inventor. Even the sharks don't argue with results!

In creating credibility with others, it's not just the results that count; it's people's awareness of the results. Thus, it's important to be able to appropriately communicate results to others, just like budding entrepreneurs do on the *Shark Tank*.

One of the strongest marketing campaigns I've seen in the optometry field is a practice that specializes in vision therapy. For those unfamiliar, vision therapy is a type of physical therapy for the eyes and brain. It involves non-surgical treatment for many common visual problems such as lazy eye, double vision, and reading and learning disabilities.

The patient base of this particular practice is predominantly children. The children are accompanied to the exam by very concerned parents. They have a very high success rate with treatment, which leads to word-of-mouth referrals by happy patients and parents, but they also showcase their results through social media.

With the parent's permission, they create video testimonials and post these on their website and social media platforms. The videos are well produced and typically involve an emotional parent discussing the life-changing impact that treatment had on their child. It's very powerful.

Many people have never heard of vision therapy, which is why I briefly described it above for those who don't work in the eye care field. Physicians who do vision therapy offer claims that it is an effective treatment for certain vision disorders, which it is. However, claims alone often fail to generate a high level of trust. Proof, in the form of results, always trumps claims.

Whatever field you are in, don't keep results hidden. Do you want to be known as the "best" in your field? You don't get to be the best at anything without delivering consistent results. If you can do that, it can be used as a tool in your marketing and branding to attract new patients, while current patients will have a higher level of trust that translates to improved clinical outcomes.

In the words of Henry Wadsworth Longfellow, "We judge ourselves by what we feel capable of doing, while others judge us by what we have already done."

WHAT'S YOUR INTENT?

It would be a huge oversight to write a chapter about trust and not mention intent. Trust is a delicate thing that's difficult to define, but we have to accept that we often find ourselves distrustful of others until they prove themselves trustworthy.

The General Social Survey reveals that only 31% of Americans believe that other people can be trusted, down from 48% three decades ago.[37]

As discussed, healthcare professionals are no exception to this. We also discussed how perception is reality. When we suspect a hidden agenda from someone or we don't believe they are acting in our best interests (real or perceived), we are suspicious about everything that person says and does.

If you are wheeled into the ER after a car accident needing emergency surgery for head trauma, I doubt anyone suspects the surgeon is not acting in your best interest. His or her job is to make you better.

However, many healthcare practices offer products and services, dare I say "sell" products and services, that don't exactly fall into this level of life-saving urgency. Chiropractors, dentists, optometrists, physical therapists, plastic surgeons, fitness trainers, and the list goes on.

As I'm writing this, I just got off the phone with a doctor who called because her associate doctor's production was much lower than hers. This is a very common issue brought up by optometry practice owners. In most cases, the associate doctor does not want to create the impression of selling to the patient. In this regard, I completely agree that any indication of "selling" to a patient will likely be received poorly. It will violate trust, and likely prevent change.

But here's the interesting part. The practice owner, whose production is much higher, does not feel like she is selling to her patients, and her patients do not feel sold to. She genuinely wants to help people with the products and service she offers! It all comes down to intent. In fact, this applies to anyone who sells anything. The good ones see it less as selling, and more of an act of service.

When your only concern is helping the other person, that person will have a higher level of trust in you. It bears repeating – people viewed as trustworthy have greater influence over others. Influence matters because you can impact someone else's life when you can get that person to change in a way that benefits them.

It's a matter of intent! We are suspicious of people whose motives we perceive to be primarily self-serving.

The Edelman Trust Barometer is an annual worldwide study comparing the amount of trust people have in four critical institutions: government, business, the media, and NGOs. Can you guess which institution comes out on top in most years and in most countries since the survey began? It's the NGOs—those private national and international not-for-profit "Non-Governmental Organizations" involved in addressing societal issues such as health, human rights, poverty, and the environment. In Gallup and other surveys comparing trust levels in various professions, can you guess who consistently comes out dead last? It's the politicians.[37]

Any idea on the primary differentiator between our perceptions of NGOs and politicians? I contend that it's a matter of intent. What are the motives and agendas of those involved? Do they really care about what's best for everyone involved? With NGOs, the motives are generally honorable and clear; the agenda is to add value to a specific, beneficial purpose or mission. With politicians, however, intent is often seen as doing what is best for the politician or for the party, but not necessarily for the whole.

Motive is your reason for doing something. It's the "why" that motivates the "what." The motive that inspires the greatest trust is genuine caring, which is why the C.O.N.N.E.C.T. Method starts with "Curiosity is Caring."

Trust is a delicate thing that can be gained or lost very easily. I once experienced a dramatic loss of trust in a matter of seconds with a healthcare professional I visited for back pain.

I hadn't been able to walk comfortably for months. I've struggled with issues related to a herniated disc for years, but this episode was particularly bad. Pain meds weren't doing the trick and it wasn't getting better on its own, like it normally did. I decided to make an appointment with a local chiropractor.

At the initial consultation, he looked at my X-ray and told me he thought it would take 30 sessions to resolve the issue. Fortunately, that was the exact number of visits I was covered for by my insurance, or at least that's what he initially thought. He wanted me to get an adjustment along with other in-office treatments three times a week. While he was going over this treatment plan, his receptionist ran into the room and said, "Doctor, his insurance only covers him for 10 visits!"

I was disappointed to hear this but prepared to discuss my out-of-pocket costs at this point. His next remark made my jaw drop. He paused for a moment, looked at his receptionist, then looked at me and said, "Well, I think we can probably do this in 10 visits."

Wait, what? A minute ago, when you thought I had better insurance coverage you said 30 visits. Now suddenly it's 10?

It felt like that old joke where a doctor gives a patient six months to live. The patient says he can't afford the bill, so the doctor gives him another six months.

In all fairness to chiropractors, I've been to others and they were all fantastic. Nevertheless, my level of trust in this particular doctor plummeted quickly. Just a moment ago I was looking at this person as someone who could help me by literally taking my pain away. Just like that, trust was gone, and I now viewed this person as someone mostly interested in maximizing my insurance benefits for his own gain.

Don't get me wrong, there's nothing wrong with seeking mutual benefit - genuinely wanting what's best for everyone involved. If you own a practice or a healthcare business, you SHOULD care about the success of the business. Understanding it's the revenues and profits that are reinvested back into the business in the form of technology, staffing, innovation, diagnostics, and so on, it's critical that any practice owner is mindful of the business side of the practice. For the reasons mentioned, I WANT my doctors to be successful!

There's also nothing wrong with wanting a great quality of life. As a consultant, this is an area I devote a lot of time for our clients. I find that many doctors who own a practice find themselves wanting more free time. They want to spend more time with their kids, take a vacation with their spouse, or just have more time for golfing or fishing.

Wanting a successful business and a great quality of life are noble and worthwhile goals, but we have to be mindful of the role of intent as it applies to our motives in treating the people we serve.

The problem with intent is that when the balance shifts in our direction, this is quickly recognized by the other person. Trust can be lost quickly, and it's very difficult to reestablish.

If we're really honest, we have to admit that sometimes our motives are not completely pure. Sometimes we approach situations with hidden agendas—even tiny ones—that keep us from being appropriately transparent with others. Sometimes we manifest behaviors that don't demonstrate caring, openness, and concern.

I see this often in the optometric profession. Offices will boldly claim that they always recommend the "best" eye wear, but never took the time to learn about the patient. They failed to be curious. Let's be really honest here. Do you always feel that your recommendations are in the *patient's* best interest? If you don't, then your recommendation may be aligned more with what's best for the practice, not the patient.

But I have a business to run!

Yes, you do, and I want you to be successful – both clinically and financially. But I also want to give you a different perspective to ponder. Try focusing your complete attention on the other person. Spend less time concerned about the success of your practice, and more time concerned about the success of your patient. Ask more questions and do more listening. Peel back the layers and uncover their deepest pain points. Treat each patient as a unique individual with his or her own unique sets of wants, needs and concerns. Deliver a message that effectively inspires patients to act on the information you provide, and continually strive to earn their trust.

If you do that, and you do it consistently, the money will take care of itself.

CHAPTER SEVEN

Conquer Objections

"Treat objections as requests for further information."
~ Brian Tracy

Getting people to say "Yes" to you is not easy, even when the information you're providing is timely and relevant. In the final two chapters I will focus on objections. This chapter will focus on people who are not necessarily saying "No" to you, but they aren't saying "Yes" either. They're giving you a hard "Maybe."

In the next chapter we'll take a deeper dive into this issue and explore the reasons people say "No" to you. We'll talk about people's reasons for avoiding change, and how to address that in a way that gets the patient to change for his or her own reasons. As you'll see, we often approach patients in a way that not only fails to inspire change, but also leads them to dig their heals into their reasons for not changing. More to come on that. For now, let's take a look at what "Maybe" sounds like.

- I'll think about it doc.
- I have to talk to my spouse first.
- Do you have any pamphlets you can give me?
- Maybe I'll do that next time.
- That sounds expensive.

To revisit a concept discussed earlier, it's often beneficial to pause periodically during the examination to ask the patient if they have any questions or concerns.

How does all of this sound to you?

Do you have any questions about what I'm telling you?

Do you agree that it would benefit you to [get this procedure, purchase this product, etc.]?

Give the patient an opportunity to object. It's ok. It's normal. Remember, the emotional side of the brain can be a Nervous Nellie when it comes to change. Change feels risky. What if this doesn't work? Do I really need this? Maybe I should think it over.

How do healthcare professionals respond to this? With information! Educate, educate, educate!

Is education important? Yes, of course it is, but it doesn't magically establish a connection between you and the patient. It doesn't guarantee the patient will act on the information you are providing. It doesn't ensure that the patient fully trusts what you are telling him or her. Knowing a lot about any topic gives you credibility but doesn't always give you enough influence to inspire people to change something.

If you want to have influence with people, you must first connect with them. Hopefully this book gives you the tools to do that.

There are also times during a presentation to a patient that you may have to reestablish that connection. Think of objections as some distortion in a radio signal. Something is said or communicated that creates some static in the message. If it's not dealt with, the "Maybe" may turn into a "No."

To further complicate things, objections are often silent. One of the reasons I suggest periodically asking patients for their feedback is to bring any objections to light. How many times have you tolerated someone trying to sell you something or get you to do something, all along nodding your head in apparent agreement with the other person? The other person thought you were fully on board, and you were looking for the nearest exit!

On a consulting call, I was once told by a group of opticians that the patients always agree with the doctor's reco- mmendations but as soon as they get to the optical they change their mind and say no to the opticians.

Never mind the doctor's recommendations, I just want what my insurance covers!

Let's think about this. Are we to assume that the patient, apparently on board with all the doctor's professional recommendations, had an epiphany in the hallway separating the exam room from the optical that caused him or her to forego the advice of the doctor?

Or, is it possible the patient never actually agreed with the doctor as suggested by the opticians?

Sure, the patient may have been on the same page with the doctor that the information provided was accurate, but at the same time had several silent objections.

I don't want to spend that much money.

My last doctor never mentioned this.

Why have I never heard of this test or procedure before?

The head nod just meant that the patient was listening. Sometimes it's just a gesture of politeness. When you provide information people will listen, but listening does not equate to a commitment to change. Sorry opticians, but the patients described above did not change their mind for you or the doctor.

Here's a hard truth about getting people to change their minds. People don't change their mind, but they will make new decisions based on new information. In the words of the great Zig Ziglar, when people say no they are saying no based on what they KNOW. Education allows us to provide more information that's important and relevant to patients, and also helps them overcome their objections.

Here is an easy way to look at objections. Objections, whether silent or verbalized, are often the patient asking "Why?" In my previous book, *But I Don't Sell*, I addressed these Why questions, drawing from research by David Hoffeld, author of *The Science of Selling: Proven Strategies to Make Your Pitch, Influence Decisions and Close the Deal*. As reinforced throughout this book, getting people to change requires good selling skills. I'll summarize these Why questions below. I'll approach this from an optometrist's perspective, but know that the same principles apply to any healthcare provider.

The three questions people need answered before changing:

1. Why do I need to change?
2. Why do I need to change now?
3. Why do I need *you* for this change?

Objection #1: Why change?

Why do I need to change my prescription doc? I'm seeing well with the glasses I have now.

Why do I need prescription sunglasses? I've never had them before and I'm doing ok.

Why do I need to switch contact lenses? I know you keep recommending those daily disposable lenses, but I'm not having any problems with these 2-week disposables. I know that I wear them for a month, but I've never had the pink eye doc!

The challenging part about the example objections above is that you may not ever hear the objection. These may just be thought bubbles that you can't see. All along the patient is bobbing his head up and down while you continue to talk "at" him. You educate. You inform. You prescribe.

Meanwhile, the patient feels talked "at" but not heard. This is the patient the opticians I mentioned earlier were talking about. The silent objection originated in the exam room; it was only verbalized in the optical.

Interestingly, I've heard more than one seasoned optician complain that doctors sometimes do more harm than good with their recommendations. This is almost always the case of a doctor breaking a lot of the rules laid out in this book. The biggest violation likely being the doctor sidestepped curiosity.

Doctor: *Are you having any problems with your vision?*

Patient: *Not really.*

Doctor: *Ok, good. At the end of the exam I'm going to recommend a lot of products and services I want you to purchase.*

Now whether or not the patient will benefit from these products and services is not the point here. The point is that the patient is not "sold" on change yet. You failed to establish a connection with the patient, you have very little if any influence, and it's unlikely the patient will buy into your recommendations.

The reason is so simple and obvious. It's the same reason you resist changing when someone else is trying to get you to do something. People change for their own reasons, not someone else's. When we do change for someone else, it often feels uncomfortable, even forced.

Imagine all your patients are wearing a T-shirt that says in bold letters, "What's in it for me?" Stop giving people all your reasons for change without taking the time to understand what's important to them. Work to uncover that answer in your questions and case history. When you can do that, the question of "Why change?" becomes easy to answer.

Objection #2: Why now?

What's the rush doc?

Can't this wait till next year?

I'll tell you what, just give me my script and I'll come back when I have more time!

In sales, it's generally accepted that the longer the sales cycle (the time between presenting a product or service and a purchase), the less likelihood of a sale. This has been demonstrated in eye care, as some studies have found that approximately 25 percent of patients who claim they will come back later to make a purchase never actually return, and the ones who do spend less money. Many of the things that you discuss and recommend to patients will be forgotten within 24 hours if not acted on.[7] Many of these patients who return several days, weeks or even months later have forgotten what you recommended and why you recommended it. "Oh yeah, I think I remember her saying something about that but I'm just going to go with what my insurance covers."

There will not always be a justification for making a change now versus later, but many times there is. How often have you recommended or prescribed a solution to a patient that you felt was in their best interest and they resisted taking action, pushing off a decision until later? Are there times when you felt it was in the patient's best interest to act sooner than later? This could be for clinical reasons or even a concern that if the patient did not follow your recommendations now, he or she may not act at all. Some examples might be the early cataract patient who pro-crastinates the purchase of prescription sunglasses, the contact lens abuser who agrees to "consider" daily disposables at his next exam, or the convergent insufficient child whose parents want to "see how things go" this year in school before agreeing to vision therapy treatment.

While it's usually not the best course of action to make the patient or consumer feel pressured into making a change, are there times when building some urgency into your message will get people to take action sooner than later? Nobody wants to feel pressured into making a change, but some people just need a nudge in the positive direction. When appropriate, help people understand why taking action now versus later is in their best interest.

If the patient is not committed to making the full change, then lower the bar for success. In reality, the urgency of our recommendations will not always be the same. It may sound counterintuitive for a healthcare professional to say this, but a lot of your patients who smoke don't need to fully kick the habit today. In fact, if you pushed them to make that change immediately, they would likely be resistant and may even try to justify their own reasons for not changing. Some momentum is better than none. Change is a process. Perhaps the goal becomes reducing the number of cigarettes smoked per day. Get the patient to agree and commit. We'll talk about this more in the next chapter.

Objection #3: Why you?

Why not the doctor across town?

Why not the big box optical?

Why not the Internet?

Why YOU?

For this objection I'm going to lean on the focus of the previous chapter, "trust." As a consumer, have you ever been in a situation where getting the best deal was your top priority? Of course you have! Some of this was a result of a knowledge gap. You lacked the knowledge and information necessary to make a decision based on value, so price became the most important factor. Perhaps this was a computer, car, health club membership, or even a new piece of equipment for your practice. But then something interesting happened. You conversed with somebody who started to fill in this knowledge gap. This may have been a representative or salesperson from the company. They asked questions. Became more familiar with your situation and how the product could benefit you based on your unique needs and interests. They also made you aware of what you would be losing by choosing the "cheapest" option. This person appeared to have a high level of knowledge about the product or service being discussed and your confidence and trust in this person increased. Based on this, you started to place more value on this person's recommendations. In fact, NOT doing business with this person began to feel... Risky!

If you're still unsure how to establish trust with your patients, go back and reread the previous chapter. Establishing trust requires some work on your part. The letters after your name and degree on the wall help, but that alone doesn't distinguish you from other practitioners in your field. If there's a business component to your practice and you have competitors marketing their services to people in your area, it's critical for the success of your practice that trust is very high.

The same applies to your current patients. In optometry, there are many options for people to receive eye care. Even when people visit an optometrist for an eye examination, they have the option of purchasing their eye wear at another optical. We're back to the question of, "Why you?"

If you have established your authority as an expert, possess exceptional capabilities beyond the average clinician in your field, and can demonstrate that you consistently produce results for patients, the question of "Why you?" becomes obvious. In the mind of the patient, the question becomes, "Why *not* you?"

HANDLING AN OBJECTION

We'll dive deeper into the area of objections in the next chapter. In that chapter we'll discuss the reasons people resist change, even when it would benefit their health, and how to effectively motivate those people to embrace change.

In the course of treating patients, a lot of minor objections may pop up that interfere with the patient's commitment and willingness to change. Below I'll suggest a quick, three-step process for addressing, and hopefully conquering, these minor objections. Remember, even a minor objection can be enough to cause the decision-making part of the brain to put up a stop sign.

Step one: Listen to the patient

At this point in the book, it's probably no surprise that I suggest more listening when the issue is an objection. Curiosity is as important as ever when a patient is objecting.

Don't interrupt. Don't interject. In fact, don't do anything other than give the patient your full attention until they are completely done talking. This alone will communicate empathy and understanding. Our knee-jerk reaction in these situations is often to jump in and tell the other person they are wrong. It's better to just agree with the patient at this point. Remember, you're just agreeing with their perception of the situation, not their position. If I say it's hot and you say it's cold, neither of us are wrong. I can agree that you think it's cold. Trying to convince someone they are wrong at this point is like swimming upstream. Most people don't drown from water in their lungs, they drown from exhaustion.

Most people are open to receiving more information, but not until they have had a chance to fully communicate their thoughts and feelings. Remember, an objection is not always a "No," it's often a request for further information. Objections are truly an opportunity for you to learn more about the patient's desires and their understanding of the issue at hand.

Step 2: Repeat their concern back to them

Whenever we object to anything, it's important to us that we feel heard. Put yourself in a position of having doubts or concerns about a product or service you are considering, and the salesperson keeps interrupting you, even looking annoyed at times with your reluctance to move forward with a purchase. Not only are you less likely to embrace additional information the salesperson could provide, but you find yourself wanting to be "right." This is not an advantageous position to be in when trying to get someone else to take action or make a change.

It's important not only to listen to the other person, but also repeat back to that person what you heard to demonstrate your understanding of their concerns. The ability to make connections is a key part of this book, and in an odd way this sometimes involves making a connection on reasons *not* to change.

That doesn't mean that you and the patient necessarily agree on not changing, but the connection comes in your ability to understand and relate to their perception of the situation. Below is an example.

Thank you for explaining your concerns to me. What I'm hearing you say is [paraphrase patient's concerns]. Is that correct?

Not only does this demonstrate that you were listening to the patient and understand his or her concerns, but it also serves as an opportunity to clear up any miscommunications or inaccuracies in the patient's understanding of the situation. Most objections fall into two categories: misunderstandings and valid objections.

Step 3: Reposition your argument for change (taking the objection into consideration)

Once you've listened to the patient's objection and repeated it back to him or her, you can now offer more information. What information you provide will vary based on the situation. It may involve clearing up a misunderstanding. It could involve delivering more information if you feel, based on the patient's comments, they don't have all the information needed to make an educated and informed decision. Make sure the information you are providing is relevant to the patient's concerns, otherwise you risk the "feature dump" scenario common in sales where a salesperson keeps presenting features hoping something will stick. The problem with a feature dump is that it often fails to connect with the consumer and essentially becomes a long list of reasons for NOT purchasing a product or service if it's not relevant to the buyer.

In many cases, the best approach is repositioning your argument for change taking the patient's objections into consideration. This may involve a concession on your part, but also presents an opportunity to shine a spotlight on something discussed in an earlier chapter – desire for gain and fear of loss. In the world of sales, these are known as dominant buying motivators. These two motivators are relevant in non-sales selling as well, getting people to act on the information they are presented with. In these cases, after following steps 1 and 2, reposition your argument for change taking the patient's concerns into consideration, but also use this opportunity to restate desire for gain and fear of loss.

Here is an example:

> *Ms. Smith. Thank you for bringing these issues to my attention. If I'm hearing you correctly, you're saying [paraphrase patient's concerns]. I do understand why that's a concern of yours. We do have other options to address this condition, but I want to remind you that alternative options won't fully address the problem you were having (desire for gain) and offer less chance of a full recovery (fear of loss).*

Restating desire for gain and fear of loss forces the patient to consider, one last time, what they are not getting or potentially giving up by not following your advice. As a practicing optometrist, I used this approach frequently when patients expressed reluctance to spend additional money on their eye care, such as a special lens coating to minimize glare or glasses specifically for occupational use.

> *Mr. Smith, thank you for bringing your concerns to my attention. I completely understand what you're saying. We can certainly go with a lower cost option if that is a concern, but I want to remind you that this may not fully resolve the problems you mentioned with computer use. You said you spend much of your working day on a computer. I think the options I recommended will provide the greatest relief from the headaches and neck pain you are experiencing (desire for gain). Are you ok if those problems persist with your new glasses (fear of loss)?*

In my experience, sometimes the patient held firm to his or her decision to avoid spending additional money on their vision. However, this approach almost always led to a moment where the patient visibly paused to consider the options. The focus of their attention moved from price to value. In the same way that a good salesperson works to create value that outweighs price, the same approach can be applied in health care by getting the patient to value the health benefits more than whatever it is he or she is objecting to. After reflecting on their options, patients would often reconsider their decision and be willing to prioritize their vision over cost.

This scenario would typically apply when a patient has multiple treatment options. You might have your preference for the patient and share that with the patient, but he or she expresses reluctance to move forward with your recommendation. There are certainly times when a clinician must be direct with patients, but there are also times when getting a patient to do *something* is better than nothing. This is the difference between a directive style and a guiding style. Both have their place in doctor – patient interactions. We'll get more into that in the next chapter.

This is a good time to recap a few things, especially for the "Who's the doctor here?" holdouts. Patients don't have to do what we say, and too often don't do what we want them to. Sometimes they bob their head in respectful agreement and then move on with their life without applying the information we've given them. It's not uncommon for patients to act on the information we've provided for a short time, and then return to their previous habits and behaviors. Remember, getting people to act on the information we provide usually requires change, and change is hard. If change is perceived as too difficult, too big, or too risky, people will often respond by not changing at all.

Could you dismiss a patient from your practice for non-compliance? Sure. I'm not disputing that there's a time to part ways with a patient. If someone is putting their health at risk, and as a result putting your professional liability and reputation at risk, you may have to inform this patient that you can no longer be their healthcare provider. However, I think we can agree that's a drastic step that would be best avoided if possible.

Before "firing" a patient for not following your advice, let's take a closer look at why people are slow to change, and how to motivate them to take action.

CHAPTER EIGHT

Tell Me What to Do

"Give people enough guidance to make the decisions
you want them to make."
- Jimmy Johnson

D on't even start lecturing me about the cigarettes!

This was a comment made to me by a patient while he was clutching a pack of Marlboro Lights in his shirt pocket. He made the comment about five minutes into the exam when I asked about his smoking habit. We were off to a great start!

Essentially, he was saying, "Don't tell me what to do!"

Recognizing I probably was not going to have any success *changing* his mind, his habits, or his health priorities at that very moment, I backed off and moved on to other questions.

DOCTOR, PLEASE TELL ME WHAT TO DO

It would be great if every patient encounter ended with the patient saying this. Sometimes they do. There are certainly times when a clinician asks questions to learn more about the patient's symptoms and concerns, provides information and insight on the patient's condition, and the patient responds with an unconditional desire and commitment to follow the physician's advice.

These patients do not require a high level of "selling" as it regards to making changes that positively benefit their health. Some people are naturally compliant with whatever their doctor suggests. Or perhaps you made such a solid case for change (the focus of this book), that the patient saw no other alternative than to follow your advice. By the time you are prescribing a solution, these patients are *pre-sold*.

Most importantly, these patients are more likely to follow through with their part, whether it's losing weight, starting an exercise program, or improving compliance with a glaucoma medication.

Fortunately, because we're highly educated and trained physicians, nearly ALL patients follow our advice and make whatever behavior changes we recommend or prescribe. After all, we're doctors!

[*Sound of car screeching*]

Ok, snap out of it. Can we once again address a huge problem in patient care? Many patients don't follow our advice. Despite repeated attempts to get patients to "change" something, many simply hear our words but fail to act on them.

In the preceding chapters I gave you practical and scientifically supported strategies for getting patients to *buy* into change. It is my sincere hope that this helps you to be more influential with the patients you serve, leading to happier patients and improved outcomes. It's also my desire that creating more clinical success will lead to a more fulfilling career for you, and also a more financially successful practice.

So why do so many patients ignore their doctor's advice? Since it's the area I'm most familiar with, let me address the issue from an optometrist's perspective. Many optometrists recommend, or train their staff to recommend, multiple pairs of eyeglasses for various uses. Everyday glasses for everyday use. Sunglasses for outdoors. Computer glasses for (you guessed it) computer use. There are even glasses for specific activities like golf and hunting.

On average, the percentage of multiple pairs sold by optometry practices is around 5 percent of total sales. It's safe to say the majority of patients are saying "no" to the doctor. The *change* in this case would be getting the patient to purchase glasses that would provide additional value and benefit to their vision and/or ocular health.

Optometrists also struggle in other areas where patients frequently decline their recommendations. Many practices strive to add specialized services, such as sports vision or vision therapy, or sell products like dry eye masks or nutritional supplements, only to have the patient say thanks, but no thanks.

If you are a doctor, nurse, physical therapist, dentist, dental hygienist, chiropractor, dietician, fitness trainer, or other healthcare professional, you probably have many conversations about behavior change in the course of your typical day. While healthcare professionals may not be *salespeople* in the traditional sense, you might find yourself feeling like a salesperson who's not very good at selling people on change.

You might also find yourself asking, *how do I get people to do what I want them to do? Do I need to educate more? Advise? Counsel? Warn?*

When it comes to getting patients to take action or make a change, there is an approach that has grown in popularity in recent years. It's called motivational interviewing, and it works by activating the patient's own motivation for change.

WHAT IS MOTIVATIONAL INTERVIEWING?

This final chapter will apply many of the principles taught in the previous chapters, but specifically focus on the area of behavior change. The subtitle of this book is *How to Make Connections, Influence Decisions, and Get Patients to Buy into Change.* My position is that if you want to have more influence with people, you have to first make a connection. Once you've established a connection and gained influence, then you'll likely have more success in getting people to implement change. While the concept is rather simple, getting people to change is not easy. If it were, I wouldn't have bothered to write a book about it, and you probably wouldn't have bothered to read it.

As a health professional, you probably have a lot of conversations with patients about behavior change. The conversations arise whenever a consultation involves the patient doing something different in the interest of their health. This can involve taking a medication regularly, flossing teeth, changing one's diet, exercising, and so on. It can also involve cutting down or quitting behaviors that are harmful to one's health, such as smoking, drug abuse, overworking or eating junk food.

Clinicians talk with patients every day about these behaviors. We provide information. We offer insight. We educate. We make an iron clad case for change, only to have many of our patients decline our advice and continue along the same path. Why is that?

In the book *Motivation Interviewing in Health Care: Helping Patients Change Behavior*, authors Stephen Rollnick, William Miller and Christopher Butler tackle this very question. Is it a lack of information? Is it ignorance? Is it disinterest?

According to the authors, ambivalence is often the reason people don't change. They want to, they are able to, they see good reasons for it, they know they need to, and then they hit that "but."

"I know I should do what you're saying, but..."

This is where clinicians and health professionals would be well suited to consider an approach that gets patients to commit to change, as opposed to committing to their reasons for *not* changing.

THE TRADITIONAL APPROACH TO PATIENT CONSULTATION

As long as patients have been seeking advice and care from healthcare professionals, there has been somewhat of an uneven power relationship between the doctor and patient. The clinician asks a series of questions and then directs that passive patient on what to do. There is often very little if any active collaborative conversation or joint decision making.

While there are certainly times when a direct approach is an effective one, research in this area has revealed that there are also limitations with this approach when it comes to getting people to change behaviors.

Let's pause to consider change in our own lives. We are bombarded by marketing messages trying to sell us on change. Buy this product so you can get that result. Purchase this service so you can solve that problem.

Other people in our lives also devote a lot of energy into getting us to change. A boss wanting us to increase our work output. A spouse wanting us to stop leaving our socks on the floor. Parents wanting their kids to eat their vegetables. Even our doctors wanting us to eat healthier and lose weight.

These are all admirable requests, but how often do we hear these messages and continue doing things the same way? We ignore most marketing messages, even when the product or service would provide value to us. Kids continue to opt for French fries over broccoli, and patients who have been warned numerous times to stop smoking continue to light up.

Sometimes we'll change because someone else wants us to do something, but when change is impactful and sustaining, it's often because we followed our own motivations. We'll listen to other people's advice, but it's often our own goals, values, concerns and aspirations that drive lasting behavior change.

In health care the information we provide is very important, but we must remember that the only person who can enact change is the patient. To get people to change, we must consider *their* motivations for change. That's the science behind motivational interviewing.

There are 4 guiding principles to motivational interviewing.

1. Resist the urge to be right, and make the patient wrong.
2. Understand and explore the patient's own motivations for change.
3. Listen with empathy.
4. Empower the patient.

Below are strategies that incorporate these four principles.

RESIST THE RIGHTING REFLEX

We have all been in positions where another person was attempting to get us to see things their way. Perhaps this was someone trying to sell you something or get you to do something they wanted you to do. Think about an argument with a friend where he or she was attempting to get you to agree with them on a certain issue. Consider a political debate with a family member or an argument over money with a spouse.

Is it safe to say that in many of these very common scenarios you held your ground? Not only did you hold your ground, but you probably repeated your reasons numerous times for why you were right, and they were wrong. In these situations, how willing were you to change your point of view and acquiesce to what the other person wanted you to do or think?

While heated debates between a doctor and patient are rare, the same scenario can play out on a more subtle level if a patient is being told to change something they are not motivated to change, at least not yet.

This is the danger in telling people what we think they should do without understanding their own motivations. This is why I focus so much of this book on being curious and asking good questions. Certainly, there are times when a directive style is appropriate. A patient presenting to the ER in cardiac arrest doesn't have many options. There is no need or time to explore the patient's motivations for emergency surgery. But there are numerous situations clinicians face every day where informing and educating without understanding the patient's motivations fails to result in the desired change.

- Stop smoking
- Lose weight
- Floss your teeth every day
- Take medications as prescribed

- Stop over-wearing contact lenses
- Return for follow-up care
- Get more sleep
- Get a yearly eye exam
- And on and on

I want to introduce the concept of TBU information. TBU stands for "true but useless." I hear doctors constantly talk about how they educate and inform patients. Certainly, that is an important responsibility of healthcare professionals, but how useful is it if it doesn't get the patient to DO something?

Let me repeat that. How useful is information if it doesn't get patients to DO what you want them to do?

The sad reality is that healthcare professionals provide true but useless information every day. Patients hear what we are saying, but it doesn't lead to meaningful results or outcomes. Patients leave our offices wiser, but don't apply the information in ways that lead to better health or desired outcomes. Let's continue to explore the concept of motivational interviewing and how it can lead to more doing.

Healthcare professionals often activate the righting reflex when attempting to correct a behavior or get the patient to change something. The patient is doing something wrong, and as their doctor we want to make it right. Although this is well-intended, if the patient is not motivated to do what the clinician is suggesting, resistance is common. While most patients aren't bold enough to argue or openly disagree with someone wearing a lab coat with a lot of degrees hanging on the wall behind them, and may even appear to be agreeing with what their doctor is saying by politely bobbing their head up and down, this does not indicate that the patient is motivated or committed to doing what their doctor is suggesting.

Whether verbally or silently, resistance sounds like this:

I hear what you're saying, BUT that's not important to me.

I know I should do that, BUT it's too expensive.

I agree with the information, BUT I'm too busy for that right now.

Here's why the righting reflex often fails to activate change. When people are told to do something for reasons that are not motivating to them, their tendency is to defend the status quo or argue against change, just like in the scenarios presented above. In fact, sometimes the righting reflex not only fails to result in change, it can actually reinforce people's reasons for *not* changing. The more people hear themselves say something, such as their reasons for not changing, the more they start to believe it and the more committed they become to maintaining the status quo.

This is where ambivalence takes hold. People see value in the information you are providing, but if it requires doing something this is not aligned with *their* motivations, they are quick to hit that "but." Just like politics, religion and even health care, if you push on the reasons for change, people become more committed to their reasons for not changing.

Motivational interviewing can be effective in these situations because the objective is to get people to voice their own argument for change. Instead of directing the patient to change something we want them to do, we are guiding them to change based on their own motivations.

PRE-COMMITMENT TALK

As discussed in chapter 4, getting a commitment from the patient to change a behavior or take an action is a more reliable predictor of change than telling the patient what we think they should do without their involvement or commitment.

Unfortunately for both the clinician and patient, there is a wide gap between ambivalence and commitment that we need to close before the patient will make the change or take the steps we are recommending.

Instead of giving the patient our reasons for change, it's often more effective to get the patient to voice his or her own reasons for change. In other words, we want to get patients to talk themselves into changing, as opposed to getting them to verbalize their argument against change which often happens when we apply the righting reflex. We want to elicit "change talk," not resistance.

Pre-commitment talk involves getting the patient to express his or her own desire, ability, reasons and need for change.

- Desire - what they want to do
- Ability - how they could do it
- Reasons - why they would change
- Need - how important it is

You can remember this as DARN. When you evoke the above, you are fueling the human desire for change. Below are a few sample questions that could be applied to a patient who smokes cigarettes.

"Why would you want to quit smoking [Desire]?"

"How would you do it, if you decided to [Ability]?"

"What are the three best reasons for quitting [Reasons]?"

"How important is it for you [Need]?"

You could apply the above questions to a wide variety of situations where changing a behavior would benefit the patient who has shown reluctance or resistance to make that change. Notice this doesn't feel pushy or intrusive. There is less chance the patient will show resistance or defensiveness, which is likely to push the patient to defend his or her reasons for NOT changing.

While these questions may not immediately trigger a change, getting patients to voice their own motivations is a good first step toward the person taking initial steps to change. Think of this like placing little weights on the pro-side of change. It tips the balance in the direction of change.

Remember, change can be anything that involves doing something different that benefits the patient's health or well-being. If you're a dentist, you want patients to start flossing daily. If you're a physical therapist, you want people to commit to doing home exercises between sessions. If you're an optometrist, you might want patients to wear special lenses in their glasses to reduce headaches and eyestrain during computer use. Health outcomes are heavily dependent on the patient's behavioral choices and doing something new or differently.

Not only is the ability to "sell" patients on change beneficial to the patient on a clinical level, it's also beneficial to the practice on a financial level.

3 CORE COMMUNICATION SKILLS

I've stressed throughout this book the value of asking good questions and being curious about the patient. Good clinician - patient conversations should be evocative in getting patients to reveal their reasons for wanting to take an action or change something that will ultimately add value to their health or well-being.

Healthcare professionals often approach patients with an ask - inform approach. Start by asking questions, then provide information. Perhaps this cycle repeats itself as the clinician asks follow-up questions, then provides additional information.

Can you see what is missing here? Listening! While it would not be fair to say there is no listening, studies have confirmed there is often a lack of listening as doctors are quick to interrupt patients. That may be due to a lack of time or a perception that we already know what is best for the patient without needing a lot of details. Regardless, this approach is more of a directing style. Find out what's wrong (ask) and then diagnose and recommend treatment (inform).

This approach tends to be neglectful of active listening. Asking questions is not listening. In fact, firing off several questions in a row can indicate you're not listening. It can demonstrate you're not reflecting on what the patient is saying.

A good guide will ask, inform and listen in that order. It's a person, not an information receptacle. Create moments of silence where the patient has a chance to express his or her thoughts and concerns. Listen for the DARN statements that elicit the patient's own motivations for change. Occasionally reflect back to the patient what you heard and understood. Agree with and support THEIR reasons for change. This is what a good guide does.

As mentioned, there are times when a directive style (ask – inform) is appropriate, however; this chapter is devoted to patients who are showing or have demonstrated a reluctance to follow your advice. Motivational interviewing involves asking people questions with a desire to learn about their motivations. When resistance is preventing action, then adopting an approach of guiding people to an outcome that is aligned with what is important to them is often more effective.

QUANTIFY THE PAIN

As a practicing optometrist, I adopted an approach of trying to uncover problems beyond "I'm here for new glasses." I realized a lot of patients would only reveal superficial information at the beginning but would reveal additional problems as the exam proceeded. What I learned to do was elicit these problems earlier by asking better questions.

I also learned that not all problems are created equal. And by problem, I'm not referring specifically to clinical conditions. Things like lifestyle, convenience and even price can be "problems" for people. The bigger the problem, the more motivated people are to find a solution.

To quantify the pain (problem) someone is experiencing, ask the patient to offer a subjective rating from 1 to 10 measuring readiness, desire or commitment to change.

"How strongly do you feel about wanting to get more exercise? On a scale from 1 to 10, where 1 is 'not at all' and 10 is 'very much', where would you rank yourself?"

If they respond with a low number, like a 3, our reaction is often corrective. Why isn't this more important to you? You should take your health more serious!

A response like this is likely to evoke defensiveness. An alternative approach aligned with the guiding style is to ask why the patient didn't pick a lower number.

"Ok, why didn't you pick a 2?"

Now, the patient has to begin thinking about why he's not a 2? He then begins articulating his own autonomous, intrinsically motivated reasons for wanting to do something.

We know from a mountain of social science research that when people have their own reasons for doing something, they're more likely to endorse the behavior and more likely to carry it out.[39] This becomes a way to surface the patient's own motivation for change by asking questions as opposed to dictating.

Another example for my optometry friends:

> Clinician: *On a scale from 1 to 10, how motivated are you to start wearing sunglasses outdoors?*
>
> Patient: *I would say 2.*
>
> Clinician: *Ok. Why didn't you say 1?*
>
> Patient: *Well, I know when I do wear sunglasses my eyes feel more relaxed outdoors. I also know that my risk of other eye problems you've told me about will reduce if I protect my eyes from the sun.*

Notice that the patient is now expressing his own reasons for behavior change. You learn not only how important the change is to a patient but also why it is important.

Another approach is to simply get the patient to discuss pros and cons. They will then verbalize their own reasons for and against change.

This requires clinicians to do something that doesn't come natural for us. It requires us to give up control over the outcomes. Giving up control down not mean a lack of influence, but granting autonomy to the patient is sometimes exactly what's needed to guide him or her to take action.

Human beings only have two responses to control. They comply or they defy.

WHAT'S NEXT?

Getting someone to express their DARN statements is a great first step, but ultimately, you need to get someone's commitment to increase the odds they will implement what you are recommending. Once the patient has expressed why they see change as important, then test their level of commitment to change.

"So, what do you make of all this now?"

"What do you think you'll do?"

"What would be a first step for you?"

The normal answers to these questions would be commitment language. The strength of their answers gives you an indication of their level of commitment. Low commitment suggests a further exploration of their DARN statements or notes in their chart to revisit the topic at subsequent visits. It's also possible that a seed is planted that prompts further contemplation by the patient in the days and weeks following the exam. Patients may do their own research on a product, service or procedure you recommended. Some patients may return wanting to discuss issues raised at a previous visit. In spite of the delay, consider that a win!

TELL ME WHAT TO DO

The direct approach to patient consultations is for the doctor to ask and then inform. Essentially, we are telling the patient what to do. That can be effective with people open to their doctor's recommendations and motivated to take action. Sometimes patients present to their doctor with this very request, "Tell me what to do." Where ambivalence exists, it's better to explore and uncover the patient's motivations for change.

Above we discussed reflective listening, where you allow for moments of silence in your interactions with patients for them to respond. This is a time for you to listen, while occasionally reflecting back to the patient what you heard. Through this process you are collecting the patient's DARN statements, commitments and next steps to deliver back to the patient as a final summary. In the book *Motivation Interviewing in Health Care*, the authors describe this as collecting a bouquet of all the reasons the patient has offered for change and presenting him or her with it. You are not directing these patients; you are guiding them.

At this point, even an ambivalent patient may look to you for direction. At some point in our lives we've all been talked into or out of something, but we likely chose a new or different path as a result of better understanding how the change would benefit us. It's at this point that we are more willing to look at someone we believe can help us and say, "Tell me what to do." We are giving the other person permission to tell us what to do.

If you sense the patient will be apprehensive or defensive about the information you intend to provide, then ask permission to offer information or advice. This lowers resistance by emphasizing the collaborative nature of the relationship.

"Can I tell you what I think will help you?"

"Can I tell you what I think you should do?"

"Can I tell you what has worked well for others?"

This is an indirect way of getting patients to grant permission for you to offer information and advice. One way or another, we need to move beyond resistance with ambivalent patients. People tend to be more open to other people's feedback when they have given them permission to grant it. Remember, the focus of this chapter is resistant patients, so the approach needs to be adjusted.

A particularly effective approach I've discovered is talking about what has worked well for others. A large part of my expertise as a doctor and later as a consultant came from the number of patients and clients I have worked with. Where people can be closed off to advice directed at them, they are typically open to hearing what has worked well for others. This avoids the righting reflex or suggesting what the patient should do. A good follow-up question can be, "Do you think it's reasonable you could attain the same results?"

If you feel that permission asking is not appropriate for a situation and you need to be more direct, you can adjust the delivery.

"There is something I need to tell you."

"I understand this may not concern you at this time, but…"

"I have some concerns I want to share with you."

Offering choices is another way to guide patients that still allows for autonomy but is more directive when the situation calls for it. This approach stops short of telling people what to do, but instead provides tailored choices.

"Since you're diabetic and at higher risk for eye disease, we can do a dilated fundus exam today or we can reschedule that."

"We can switch you to a different brand of contact lenses that allows more oxygen to your eyes or we can take a break from wearing contact lenses."

Offering multiple choices at a time and asking the patient to choose avoids the patient arguing for the reasons against change when only one option is presented.

THE KNOW-IT-ALL PATIENT

Occasionally we have the privilege of examining Mr. or Ms. Know-It-All. You know the one. These are the patients who question the medical advice they receive from a health professional but believe everything they read on the Internet. One study found that over half of millennials believe the information they find online is "as reliable" as their doctor.[40]

Not to pick on millennials. I experienced this many times with other age groups as well. One of my more memorable encounters was a patient at high risk for glaucoma who brushed off my concerns by saying, "I know I can't have glaucoma because I smoke a lot of pot."

In my experience, the know-it-all patients can be especially resistant to information that doesn't align with their preconceived notions. Instead of activating the righting reflex, use this opportunity to open knowledge gaps by asking them to discuss their understanding about the condition.

"So I don't concentrate on the wrong things, tell me what you already know about diabetic retinopathy?"

The answer you get back may reveal they actually do understand the condition, but this also allows you to both open and fill knowledge gaps. As you provide information, pause and ask the patient to interpret it.

"What are some things you can do to control your blood sugar level?"

Agree where appropriate. Comment on their knowledge. Ask permission to give information that may differ or contradict their current understanding.

"Can I offer a few suggestions that may help you do an even better job?"

"Can I share some information with you that you may not be aware of?"

"Can I tell you what many of my other patients have done to avoid diabetic vision loss?"

There is an art to communication and conveying information in an effective way. It's not a perfect science and will require some experimentation and trial and error on your part. You may need to adjust your approach if the patient appears disconnected, defensive or defiant. On the other hand, if you feel a connection with the patient, the patient appears engaged with what you are saying, and is asking questions about how he or she might make the change you are recommending, then you know you are on the right track.

Patients need direction from doctors, but this doesn't mean they always do what we suggest. Ambivalence often stems from not seeing something as important, or not weighing the outcome of change greater than the outcome of maintaining the status quo. When motivational interviewing is effective, a light switch is flipped, and patients make the decision that it really is important.

People naturally resist change and telling people what to do before they're ready to hear it can be woefully ineffective in getting people to take action. It's much more effective when you are talking to a captive audience. When someone understands how you can help them, they will not only be ready to hear what you have to say, they will *want* to hear what you have to say.

Ultimately, this is where we need to get patients if we want them to change. Make a connection, gain influence, and get patients to open their mind to change. It's at this point where a patient, even one previously resistant to doing what you recommended, will look to you and say…

"Tell me what to do."

Back to my chain-smoking patient who didn't want to be lectured on cigarettes. I would best describe him as someone with a rough exterior. He didn't look like someone who smiled often, and cantankerous would be a good description of his demeanor. He was in his late 50s and had several health conditions, including hypertension. I discovered something during the examination that forced me to revisit the smoking topic. He had bleeding in the back of his eyes from a condition called hypertensive retinopathy. Smoking may have not been the only cause, but it certainly wasn't helping. He did agree to see a specialist about the condition. I told him he needed to address the bleeding before we could get an accurate glasses prescription, and asked him to return once he was released by the ophthalmologist.

Several weeks later I walked into the same exam room and he was waiting to be seen. The person who returned was not the same person who originally sat down in the chair and demanded we not discuss his cigarette habit. His body language was softer. He spoke with less defiance. He actually appeared happy to see me.

We talked. He shared stories about his life. He told me about his kids and how he recently became a grandpa. His wife had passed recently and his family meant everything to him. The thought of losing his vision and not being able to enjoy seeing his kids and playing with his grandkids was unthinkable for him. These were *his* reasons for wanting to change.

Through tears, he looked at me and said, "Tell me what to do."

Conclusion

In 2005, an article was published in Fast Company entitled "Change or Die." The article presented studies conducted with patients who had severe medical conditions that required lifestyle changes in order to live. After only 12 months, 90 percent of the patients had reverted back to their old lifestyles, virtually guaranteeing an impending death.[41]

Change is hard. If we are going to effectively impact the patients we serve, we need to change as well.

Recently I was talking with a colleague who specializes in dry eye disease and lectures nationally on the topic. He developed a boot camp for other doctors wanting to implement this specialty into their practice. He told me that his motivation for continuing to offer this boot camp and offer it in multiple cities was that he saw "behavior change" in the clinicians who attended. He told me that without behavior change, he wouldn't have continued to offer this boot camp.

That was very refreshing to hear. I suspect many paid speakers simply show up, do their presentation, then go home and cash their check. But what impact did the speaker have on those listening if they didn't do anything with the information? What if they didn't improve some area of their life? What if they didn't execute? What if they didn't change?

I use this example to stress the point that if we want to motivate change in patients, the change needs to start with us. This book is focused on getting patients to change, but here's the rub. You have to change first. Nothing happens until you start doing something different as a clinician. The results you're getting from both a professional and financial level are a direct reflection of what you've been doing. Maybe you're doing great. Keep it up! Maybe there are some areas you could improve on. Start today. But do start.

Why do you want to be an optometrist? That's where we started this book. Why did you want to become a healthcare provider in whatever field you are in? Did you want to help people? Did you want to improve lives? Did you want to make an impact?

If you feel frustrated at times with the results and outcomes you are getting, both clinically and financially, rest assured you're not alone. I hope this book gives you the tools to better connect with patients, gain more influence over their health decisions, and get more patients to buy into change.

If you've been a healthcare professional long enough, I will bet you've had at least a few patients give you a hug and say thank you. I'll bet that their motivation for doing this was not based on information or education you provided. It was more than that. Whether big or small, you made an impact on that person. They did more than just listen to you, they took action, and they are better for it. Sharing information does not elicit this level of gratitude and emotion from the people we serve. Something had to change.

I've offered several quotes throughout this book, so I'll close with a quote of my own. Consider this food for thought, but also a bit of a challenge to make changes to your own approach to patient care that will translate into more impactful outcomes for your patients.

"If nothing changes, did you really make an impact?"

References

1. Pink, D. (2013). *To Sell is Human: The Surprising Truth About Moving Others.* Riverhead Books.
2. Khalil, S. (2018, December 21). "New Year's Resolutions Last Exactly This Long." *New York Post.* Retrieved from https://nypost.com/2018/12/21/new-years-resolutions-last-exactly-this-long/
3. Soon, CS., Brass, M., Heinze, H., & Haynes, J. (2008, April 13). "Unconscious Determinants of Free Decisions in the Human Brain." Nature Neuroscience
4. Damasio, A. (2005). *Descartes' Error: Emotion, Reason and the Human Brain.* Penguin Books
5. O'Connor, C. (2017, April 10). "Earning Power: Here's How Much Top Influencers Can Make on Instagram and YouTube." *Forbes.* Retrieved from https://www.forbes.com/sites/clareoconnor/2017/04/10/earning-power-heres-how-much-top-influencers-can-make-on-instagram-and-youtube/#7a9974e524db
6. Heath, C., Heath, D. (2010). *Switch: How the Change Things When Change is Hard.* Crown Business.
7. Renvoise, P. (2007). *Neuromarketing: Understanding the Buy Buttons in Your Customer's Brain.* Harper Collins Leadership.

8. Brooks, AW., John, L. (2018). "The Surprising Power of Questions." *Harvard Business Review.* Retrieved from https://hbr.org/2018/05/the-surprising-power-of-questions

9. Simpson, J. (2017). "Finding Brand Success in the Digital World." *Forbes.* Retrieved from https://www.forbes.com/sites/forbesagencycouncil/2017/08/25/finding-brand-success-in-the-digital-world/#601b2bb2626e

10. Interrante, A. (2018). "Doctors Interrupt Patients, Stop Listening After 11 Seconds on Average, Study Says." Newsweek. Retrieved from https://www.newsweek.com/doctor-patient-visits-1035514

11. Beckman HB, Frankel RM. Annals of Internal Medicine. 5. Vol. 101. 1984. The effect of physician behavior on the collection of data; pp. 692–696.

12. Hoffeld, D. (2016). *The Science of Selling: Proven Strategies to Make Your Pitch, Influence Decisions, and Close the Deal.* Penguin Publishing Group.

13. Charmel PA, Frampton SB. Healthcare Financial Management. 3. Vol. 62. 2008. Building the business case for patient-centered care; pp. 80–85.

14. Epstein RM, Fiscella K, Lesser CS, Stange KC. Health Affairs (Millwood). 8. Vol. 29. 2010. Why the nation needs a policy push on patient-centered health care; pp. 1489–1495.

15. Fremont AM, Cleary PD, LeeHargraves J, Rowe RM, Jacobson NB, Ayanian JZ. Journal of General Internal Medicine. 12. Vol. 16. 2001. Patient centered processes of care and long-term outcomes of myocardial infarction; pp. 800–808.

16. Radwin LE, Cabral HJ, Wilkes G. Research in Nursing & Health. 1. Vol. 32. 2009. Relationships between patient-centered cancer nursing interventions and desired health outcomes in the context of the health care system; pp. 4–17.

17. Best Care at Low Cost: The Path to Continuously Learning Health Care in America. (NCBI, 2013).

18. Lee CN, Dominik R, Levin CA, Barry MJ, Cosenza C, O'Connor AM, Mulley AG Jr, Sepucha KR. Health Expectations. 3. Vol. 13. 2010a. Development of instruments to measure the quality of breast cancer treatment decisions; pp. 258–272.

19. Johnson FR, Hauber B, Ozdemir S, Siegel CA, Hass S, Sands BE. Journal of Managed Care Pharmacy. 8. Vol. 16. 2010. Are gastroenterologists less tolerant of treatment risks than patients? Benefit-risk preferences in Crohn's disease management; pp. 616–628.

20. Street RL Jr, Haidet P. Journal of General Internal Medicine. 1. Vol. 26. 2011. How well do doctors know their patients? Factors affecting physician understanding of patients' health beliefs; pp. 21–27.

21. Fox, S. (2011). Health topics: 80% of Internet users look up health information online. Washington, DC: Pew Research Center.

22. Motor Vehicle Crash Deaths: How is the US Doing? (CDC, 2016).

23. Landro, L. (2017). "How doctors are getting more patients involved in their own care." MarketWatch. Retrieved from https://www.marketwatch.com/story/how-doctors-are-getting-patients-more-involved-in-their-own-care-2017-04-05

24. Golomb BA, McGraw JJ, Evans MA, Dimsdale JE. Drug Safety. 8. Vol. 30. 2007. Physician response to patient reports of adverse drug effects: Implications for patient-targeted adverse effect surveillance; pp. 669–675.

25. Peoples, D. (1992). *Presentations Plus*. Wiley, John and Sons, Incorporated.

26. Grimes, W. "In War Against No-Shows, Restaurants Get Tougher." New York Times. Retrieved from www.nytimes.com/1997/10/15/dining/in-war-againstno-shows-restaurants-get-tougher.html?pagewanted=all.

27. Cialdini, R. (2006). *Influence: The Psychology of Persuasion.* Harper Business.

28. Kouyoumdjian, H. (2012). "Learning Through Visuals." Psychology Today. Retrieved from https://www.psychologytoday.com/us/blog/get-psyched/201207/learning-through-visuals

29. Beck, J. (2018). "Why We Forget Most of the Books We Read." The Atlantic. Retrieved from https://www.theatlantic.com/science/archive/2018/01/what-was-this-article-about-again/551603/

30. Heath, C., Heath, D. (2007). *Made to Stick: Why Some Ideas Survive and Others Die.* Random House Publishing Group.

31. Phillips, D. (2017). The Magical Science of Storytelling (TedXStockholm). Retrieved from https://www.youtube.com/watch?v=Nj-hdQMa3uA&t=516s

32. Kramer, A., Guillory, J., Hancock, J. (2014). "Experimental evidence of massive-scale emotional contagion through social networks." Proceedings of the National Academy of Sciences of the United States of America. Retrieved from https://www.pnas.org/content/111/24/8788

33. Bedor, L. "What Makes People Like and Dislike Their Doctors?" Zocdoc: The Script. Retrieved from https://thescript.zocdoc.com/what-really-motivates-positive-and-negative-patient-reviews/

34. Carroll, A. (2015). "To Be Sued Less, Doctors Should Consider Talking to Patients More." New York Times. Retrieved from https://www.nytimes.com/2015/06/02/upshot/to-be-sued-less-doctors-should-talk-to-patients-more.html

35. Wolfson, D. (2019). "Commentary: Erosion of trust threatens essential element of practicing medicine." Modern Healthcare. Retrieved from https://www.modernhealthcare.com/opinion-editorial/commentary-erosion-trust-threatens-essential-element-practicing-medicine

36. Birkhäuer, J., Gaab, J., Kossowsky, J., Hasler, S., Krummenacher, P., Werner, C., Gerger, H. (2017). "Trust in the health care professional and health outcome: A meta-analysis." PLOS. Retrieved from https://journals.plos.org/plosone/article?id=10.1371/journal.pone.0170988

37. Covey, S. (2008). *The Speed of Trust: The One Thing That Changes Everything.* Free Press.

38. Rollnick, S., Miller, W., Butler, C. (2007). *Motivational Interviewing in Health Care: Helping Patients Change Behavior.* The Guilford Press.

39. Ferris, T. (2018). "How to Make Better Decisions and Be More Creative." *The Tim Ferris Show.* Episode #305. Retrieved from https://tim.blog/?s=daniel+pink

40. Harpaz, J. (2019). "6 Expectations Millennials Have for Their Healthcare." Forbes. Retrieved from https://www.forbes.com/sites/joeharpaz/2019/08/26/6-expectations-millennials-healthcare/#4d1c00f430ec

41. Deutschman, A. (2005). "Change or Die." Fast Company. Retrieved from https://www.fastcompany.com/52717/change-or-die

About the Author

Steve Vargo, OD, MBA is a 1998 graduate of the Illinois College of Optometry. In 2014 he joined Prima Eye Group (now IDOC) as Vice President of Optometric Consulting. A published author and speaker with 15 years of clinical experience, he now serves as IDOC's Optometric Practice Management Consultant. Since transitioning to a full-time practice management consultant, Dr. Vargo has performed over 3,000 consultations and coaching sessions with hundreds of independent optometry practices across the country. He speaks regularly at industry conferences, has been published in numerous industry publications, has a regular column in Optometric Management titled "The CEO Challenge", and is a contributing author to the widely read "Optometric Management Tip of the Week" article. Dr. Vargo has also authored 3 books on the subjects of staff management, leadership, and selling.

Dr. Vargo's other books (available on Amazon):

Eye on Management: Step-by-step guide to optometry's most common staff management challenges

Eye on Leadership: An optometrist's game plan for creating a motivated and empowered team

But I Don't Sell: An Eye Care Professional's Guide to Being More Persuasive, Influential and Successful

Questions or Comments?

I'd love to hear your thoughts. Email me at:
steve@drstevevargo.com.

NEED HELP?

I offer consulting services to independent eye care practices
through IDOC. I'll help you CHANGE your practice for
the better. Learn more at www.IDOC.net.

If this book inspired you to make a greater impact on the
lives of the patients you serve, please pass it on to someone
you want to inspire.

www.ingramcontent.com/pod-product-compliance
Lightning Source LLC
Chambersburg PA
CBHW030618220526
45463CB00004B/1341